Infertility, Assisted Reproductive Technologies and Hormone Assays

Edited by Dhastagir Sultan Sheriff

Published in London, United Kingdom

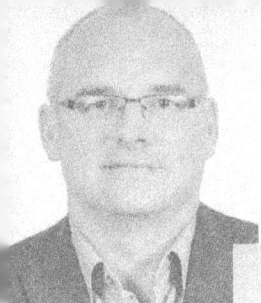
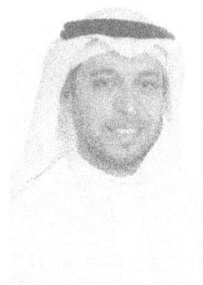
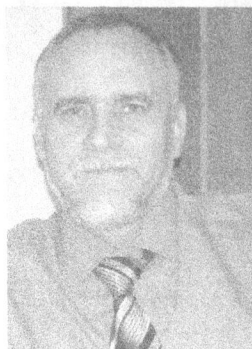
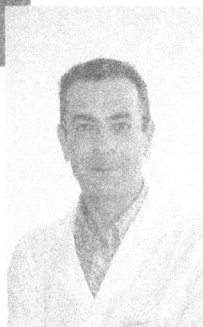
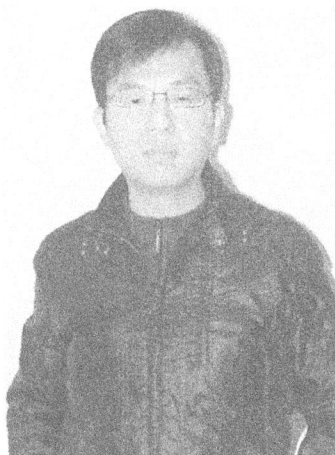
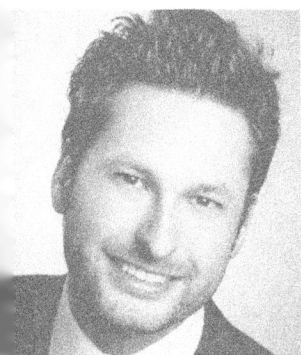
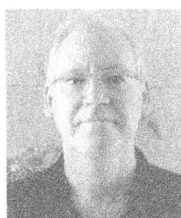

IntechOpen

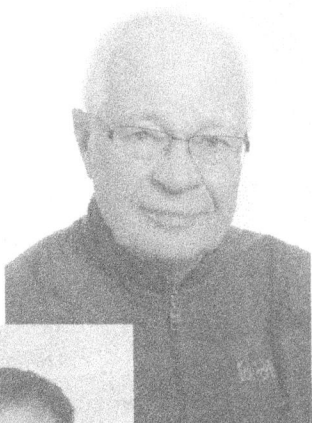
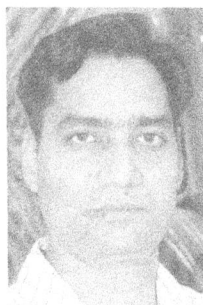
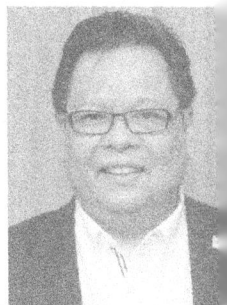
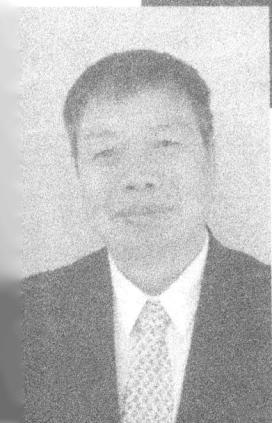
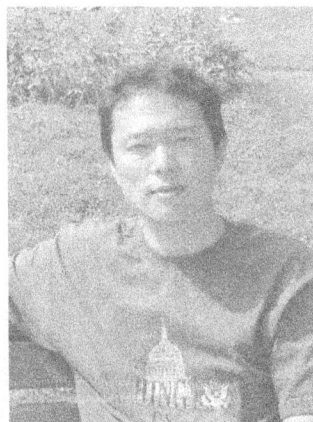
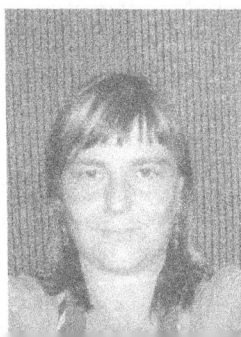

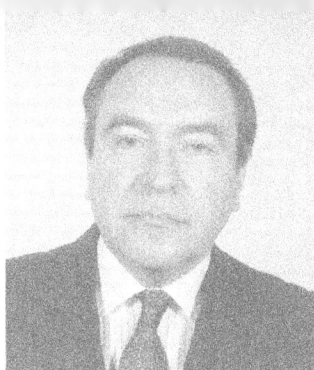

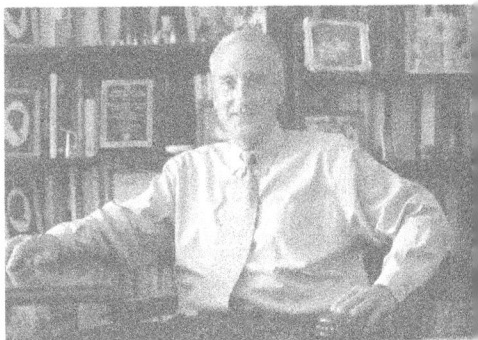

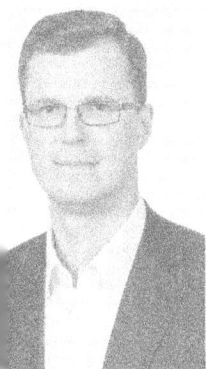

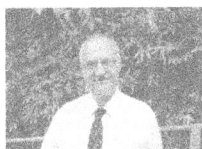

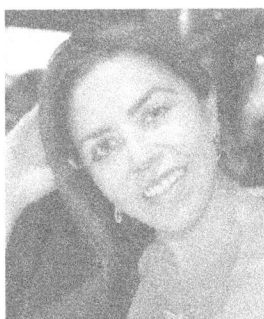

Supporting open minds since 2005

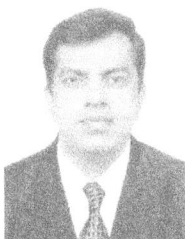

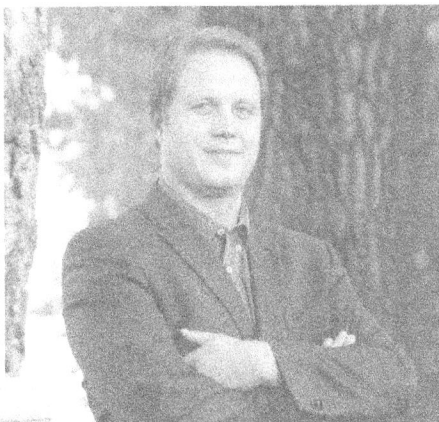

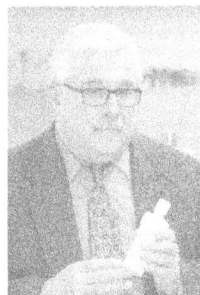

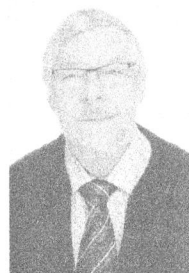

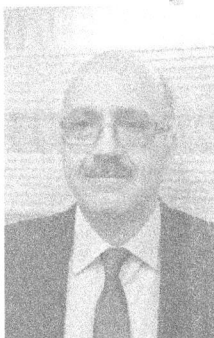

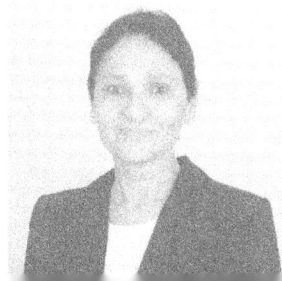

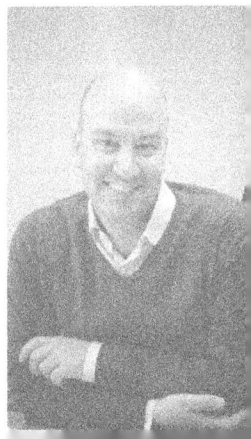

Infertility, Assisted Reproductive Technologies and Hormone Assays
http://dx.doi.org/10.5772/intechopen.73962
Edited by Dhastagir Sultan Sheriff

Contributors
Mehmet Musa Aslan, Cicek Hocaoglu, Jessica Gorgui, Anick Bérard, Arindam Dhali, Atul P Kolte, Ashish Mishra, Sudhir C Roy, Raghavendra Bhatta, Dhastagir Sultan Sheriff

Notice
Statements and opinions expressed in the chapters are these of the individual contributors and not necessarily those of the editors or publisher. No responsibility is accepted for the accuracy of information contained in the published chapters. The publisher assumes no responsibility for any damage or injury to persons or property arising out of the use of any materials, instructions, methods or ideas contained in the book.

First published in London, United Kingdom, 2019 by IntechOpen
IntechOpen is the global imprint of INTECHOPEN LIMITED, registered in England and Wales, registration number: 11086078, The Shard, 25th floor, 32 London Bridge Street
London, SE19SG – United Kingdom
Printed in Croatia

British Library Cataloguing-in-Publication Data
A catalogue record for this book is available from the British Library

Additional hard and PDF copies can be obtained from orders@intechopen.com

Infertility, Assisted Reproductive Technologies and Hormone Assays
Edited by Dhastagir Sultan Sheriff
p. cm.
Print ISBN 978-1-83881-135-8
Online ISBN 978-1-83881-136-5
eBook (PDF) ISBN 978-1-83881-137-2

We are IntechOpen,
the world's leading publisher of
Open Access books
Built by scientists, for scientists

4,200+
Open access books available

116,000+
International authors and editors

125M+
Downloads

Our authors are among the

151
Countries delivered to

Top 1%
most cited scientists

12.2%
Contributors from top 500 universities

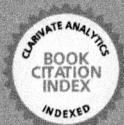

CLARIVATE ANALYTICS
BOOK
CITATION
INDEX
INDEXED

WEB OF SCIENCE™

Selection of our books indexed in the Book Citation Index
in Web of Science™ Core Collection (BKCI)

Interested in publishing with us?
Contact book.department@intechopen.com

Numbers displayed above are based on latest data collected.
For more information visit www.intechopen.com

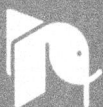

Meet the editor

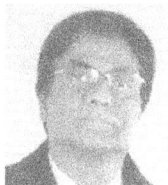

Dhastagir Sultan Sheriff received his master's and doctoral degrees in Medical Biochemistry in 1971 and 1977, respectively, from Madras Medical College in Chennai, India. Devoted to teaching, Dr. Sheriff has taught in medical schools for 35 years and visited 45 countries while doing so. He has attended 46 international conferences and organized two international conferences in medical ethics in India. He is a lifetime member of the European Society for Human Reproduction and Early Human Development; a member of the American Association of Clinical Chemistry, the Association of Physiologists and Pharmacologists of India, and the National Academy of Medical Sciences in New Delhi; and a resource person for UNESCO for Medical and Bioethics. Dr. Sheriff has authored five books including a textbook on medical biochemistry with additional interest in human sexology. He has published editorials in the *British Journal of Sexology*, *Journal of Royal Society of Medicine*, and *Postgraduate Medical Journal*. He is a scientist, former Rotarian, and Citizen Ambassador and was selected for a Ford Foundation Fellowship.

Contents

Preface   XI

Chapter 1   1
Infertility, Assisted Methods of Reproduction and Hormonal Assays
by Dhastagir Sultan Sheriff

Chapter 2   9
Medically Assisted Reproduction and the Risk of Adverse Perinatal Outcomes
by Jessica Gorgui and Anick Bérard

Chapter 3   33
Oocyte Donation
by Mehmet Musa Aslan

Chapter 4   49
Cryopreservation of Oocytes and Embryos: Current Status and Opportunities
by Arindam Dhali, Atul P. Kolte, Ashish Mishra, Sudhir C. Roy
and Raghavendra Bhatta

Chapter 5   65
The Psychosocial Aspect of Infertility
by Cicek Hocaoglu

Preface

Infertility is a major public health concern in developing and developed nations. In certain societies infertility carries a social stigma and is one of the key factors for breakup of families. The revolution created by assisted reproductive technologies (ART) in infertility treatment has given hope to many people. The quality of diagnosis plays an important role in helping to deliver proper therapy to those individuals or couples struggling with infertility. Therefore diagnostic tests and their interpretations play a vital role. Andrologists and gynecologists have helped to identify and guide patients to the proper treatment of infertility. Hormonal assays, hormonal stimulation, retrieval of healthy follicles, in vitro fertilization, and implantation and growth of embryos require a team of experts to coordinate, advocate, and advance treatment. The promising field of stem cell therapy and storage banks for sperm, oocytes, and embryos have opened new avenues of treatment and galvanized the field of reproduction. This book reviews, relates, and redeems the field of infertility treatment. It also discusses the ethical concerns related to ATR, including existing dilemmas and psychological concerns of patients.

The introductory chapter by Dhastagir Sultan Sheriff gives a bird's eye view of infertility, assisted methods of reproduction, diagnosis, and therapy, with a short note on sperm banks.

The chapter on assisted reproductive technologies and adverse outcomes by Gorgui Jessica deals with recent trends regarding the use of medically assisted methods of reproduction and perinatal outcomes, which include cognitive effects of ART.

The chapter on oocyte donation by Aslan Mehmet explains the nature, protocol, and present trends of the field. Oocyte donation is one of the necessary arms of ART. It is usually recommended for women with poor ovarian reserve possibly due to primary or secondary ovarian failure. It can be due to surgical causes, damage following chemotherapy or radiotherapy, or certain genetic disorders associated with gonadal dysgenesis, like Turner syndrome. It is reported that oocyte donation is one of the most successful techniques resulting in pregnancy, particularly in perimenopausal women.

The chapter on cryopreservation of oocytes and embryos by Dhali Arindam discusses the technique, evolution, and development of cryopreservation to benefit infertile patients. Cryopreservation of oocytes and embryos involves appreciating the multiple contexts in which cryopreservation may be applied. The chapter enables one to understand the relative impact of cryopreservation on the quality of oocytes and embryos. It allows the reader to grasp the concept of selection/attrition as it applies to the efficiency of ART. It also provides insights into the relative balance of advantages and disadvantages associated with oocyte and embryo cryopreservation in different clinical conditions. **The chapter on Cryopreservation of Oocytes and Embryos** by Dhali Arindam discusses the technique, evolution and the development to benefit human infertile patients.

Finally, the chapter on psychosocial aspects of infertility by Prof. Hocaogu Cleek explains the psychosocial domains of care in an infertility patient. One of the earlier concerns was how to incorporate psychosocial care into the infertility treatment protocol. The chapter discusses taking patient preferences and needs into account, which most often include wanting a good interaction with staff, receiving continuous care from the same doctor, receiving information that is understandable, and having a good relationship with the clinic and healthcare personnel. **The chapter on Psychosocial aspects of infertility by Prof. Hocaogu Cleek** explains the psychosocial domains of care in an infertility patient.

Dr. Dhastagir Sultan Sheriff
Reprolabs,
Chennai, India

Faculty of Medicine,
Benghazi University,
Benghazi, Libya

Chapter 1

Infertility, Assisted Methods of Reproduction and Hormonal Assays

Dhastagir Sultan Sheriff

Abstract

Infertility is a major public health concern in developing and developed nations. In certain societies, infertility carries a social stigma and is one of the key factors for breakup of families. The revolution created by assisted reproductive technologies (AIR) in infertility treatment has given hope to childless couples to have children. The quality of diagnosis plays an important role in helping to deliver proper therapy to such couples. Therefore, judicious use of diagnostic tests and its interpretation play a vital role in infertility treatment. The presence of andrologists and gynecologists has helped to identify and guide the patient to take proper treatment for their childlessness. Hormonal assays, its interpretation followed by hormonal stimulation, retrieval of healthy follicle, in vitro fertilization, implantation and growth of embryos require a team of experts to co-ordinate, advocate and advance the treatment to the patient. The promising field of stem cell therapy and storage banks of sperm, oocytes and embryos have opened new avenues of treatment and galvanized the field of reproduction. Therefore, books related to these aspects will help review, relate and redeem the field of infertility treatment. The ethical concerns of AIR will allow for introspection of the existing dilemmas and psychological concerns of the patient.

Keywords: reproductive health, infertility, assisted reproductive methods (AIR)

1. Introduction

"Health is defined as a state of physical, mental and social well-being of an individual, not merely the absence of disease" (WHO) [1–3].

It includes reproductive health with an ability to have a fulfilling sexual life, an inherent capacity to procreate with a freedom to make choices of timing and planning child birth. It also provides the couple the freedom to seek treatment modalities for family planning as well for infertility.

Infertility is one of the major reproductive health problems that challenge the clinicians as well as the couples. Another domain of reproductive health is the culture of a couple who apart from longing to have children face social pressures to beget children. In certain cultures, it carries social stigma as well as forms the basis for divorce bringing in the legal as well as ethical issues. The psychological domain acts negatively on fertility potential of the couple [4].

An added issue is gender bias and discrimination which falters the women as the major cause of infertility though science states that there are equal causes for infertility for both men and women [3].

2. Infertility

Infertility can be defined as the inability to conceive after one full year of regular, normal sexual intercourse without the use of any contraception. Infertility is a major health problem that affects a sizeable population in the world and the cause may be the male or female, with more or less 30–40% being due to the male factor or around 50% due to the female factor [5–7].

Oligospermia, poor semen quality, low sperm motility, anatomical defects like block in vas deferens, infections leading to inflammation of seminal vesicles, epididymis or prostate, genetic abnormalities like Klinefelter syndrome could represent major causes of male infertility [5–7].

Irregular ovulation, poor oocyte quality, blocked fallopian tubes due to infection or endometriosis are some of the causes of female infertility. Polycystic ovaries, primary and secondary amenorrhea, pelvic inflammatory disease (PID) and hostile cervical mucus may be less common causes of female infertility apart from cancer chemotherapy [6, 7].

2.1 Assisted methods of reproduction (ART)

35 years of assisted reproductive technology (ART) use has become one of the standard procedure of infertility treatment. More than 5 million babies are born after ART (1–5% births). Therefore, it is necessary to monitor, evaluate and trace the modifications of procedures with growing technical development of medical practice in the field of reproductive medicine [8].

Assisted reproduction techniques (ARTs) are defined as "all treatments or procedures that include the in vitro handling of both human oocytes and sperm or embryos for the purpose of establishing a pregnancy" [8].

2.2 Ovulation induction

Ovulation induction is useful in women with anovulatory or irregular ovulatory cycles. A hormone medication in tablet or injection form is administered to stimulate the production of follicle stimulating hormone (FSH). FSH then will help in the development of one or more follicles. Another hormone will then be administered to cause the release of ovum. The couples will be advised to have sexual intercourse during this period, creating a greater chance for conception [9].

2.3 Artificial insemination (AIH)

Artificial insemination (AIH) is also known as intrauterine insemination (IUI). AIH is recommended in cases of unknown etiology in women with healthy fallopian tubes or in men with erectile dysfunction or mechanical trauma which may hamper normal intercourse with the women. In certain cases before cancer chemotherapy or due to other reasons, semen stored in the sperm bank may be used for AIH [10].

2.4 In vitro fertilization (IVF)

In vitro fertilization (IVF) is a process in which ovum and sperm are allowed to fertilize in vitro. The process involves retrieval of ovum from the women and semen from the male. If successful, the embryo is then implanted in the uterus of the woman using embryo transfer [11].

2.5 Gamete intra fallopian transfer (GIFT)

The ovum is retrieved from the woman and inserted between the layers of sperm and inserted into the fallopian tube. This allows natural fertilization. It is mostly used in conditions where religious beliefs do not permit IVF [11].

2.6 Intracytoplasmic sperm injection (ICSI)

Intracytoplasmic sperm injection (ICSI) is usually done in patients with oligospermia or with abnormal semen quality. It involves direct injection of single spermatozoa into the ovum to promote fertilization [12].

2.7 Zygote intrafallopian transfer (ZIFT)

Zygote intrafallopian transfer (ZIFT) involves the transfer of zygote [13].

2.8 Preimplantation genetic diagnosis (PGD)

Preimplantation genetic diagnosis (PGD) is useful in patients with a family history of genetic disorders. It may be recommended in couples with repeated miscarriages or failure in IVF or in elder patients say 35 years old or above [14].

Aneuploidy is a term used to describe an abnormality in chromosome number (fewer or more of a specific chromosome). Aneuploidy screening is performed in cases of advanced maternal age, repeated IVF failure, recurrent miscarriage and previous aneuploidy pregnancy [15].

2.9 In vitro maturation (IVM)

In vitro maturation of oocyte-cumulus complexes is a promising new technique by which immature oocytes from small follicles less than 10 mm are matured during 30–40 h in a specific culture medium. Meta-phase II (M II) oocytes with normal morphology were inseminated by ICSI [16].

3. Making a correct diagnosis

The techniques involved in infertility diagnosis include ultrasound, computerized tomography scan (CT-scan), nuclear magnetic resonance (NMR), hysteroscopy, hysterosalpingography, laparoscopy, blood karyotyping histopathology of reproductive tissues, microbiology, serology and hormone analyses [17].

For males, standard semen analyses will be carried out to assess the sperm density, motility, fertilizing ability, and detection of anti-sperm antibodies.

Computerized analyses of semen (image analyses CASA) nowadays is used for semen analyses. Therefore, poor semen quality or primary or secondary causes of infertility (hormonal imbalance at the pituitary or at the target organ level or secondary hormonal causes like thyroid dysfunction) or even obesity will help determine and evaluate the patient for IVF or ICSI procedures [18, 19].

The treatment for infertility is judiciously adopted by the treating gynecologist at different levels by initially evaluating natural menstrual history of the patient followed by advising the couple to have sexual intercourse during the ovulatory phase. If it fails, mild ovarian stimulation with hormones will be suggested and followed by sexual intercourse. The next level of treatment may be superovulation with hormonal stimulation and retrieval of oocytes for IVF. The extra embryos or oocytes are stored for future use [19, 20].

4. Oocyte donation

Oocyte donation is one of the necessary arms of ART. It is usually recommended for women with poor ovarian reserve possibly due to primary and secondary ovarian failure. It can be due to surgical causes, damage following chemotherapy or radiotherapy, with certain genetic disorders associated with gonadal dysgenesis like Turner syndrome or patient with a known genetic disorder. It is reported that oocyte donation is one of the most successful techniques resulting in pregnancy, particularly in perimenopausal women.

One of the earlier concerns was how to *incorporate psychosocial care* into the infertility treatment protocol. This incorporation of psychosocial care is to provide the best possible care to the infertile patient. After incorporating the psychosocial care into the treatment protocol, the patient's preferences and needs are evaluated. The patient wishes to have good interaction with the staff; wishes continuity of care from the same doctor, get information that could be easily understood by the patient and to have a long standing interaction with clinic and the healthcare personnel.

Singleton pregnancies, preterm delivery and perinatal mortality as well as maternal complications, such as preeclampsia, gestational diabetes, placenta previa, placental abruption and cesarean delivery are some of the reported outcomes of ART. The following figure (**Figure 1**) explains the possible factors that may influence pregnancy outcome following ART.

Cryopreservation of oocytes and embryos involves appreciating the multiple contexts in which oocyte and embryo cryopreservation may be applied. It will enable one to understand the relative impact of cryopreservation on oocytes and embryo quality. It will allow the reader to have a grasp of the concept of selection/attrition

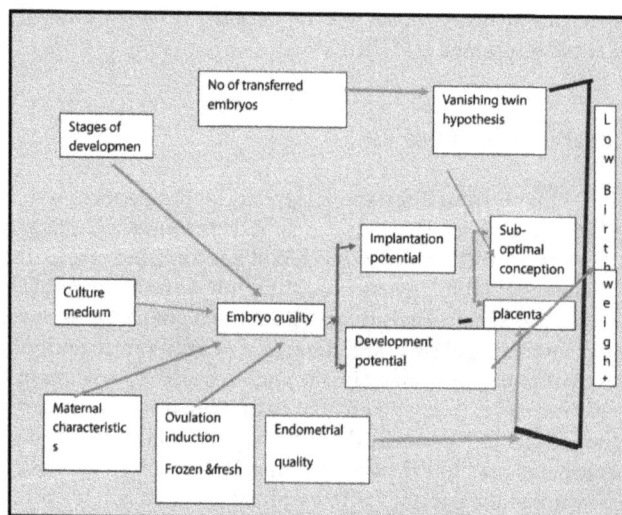

Figure 1.
The factors that affect embryo/quality which determines the outcome of assisted reproductive methods.

as it applies to the efficiency of assisted methods of reproduction (ART). It will allow to gain insights into relative balance of advantages and disadvantages associated with oocyte and embryo cryopreservation in different clinical conditions.

Apart from discussions on the nature of infertility and the assisted methods of reproduction, there are widespread discussions regarding the ethical aspects related to infertile patients and ART.

Sperm banks have become one of the accessory health centers of assisted reproductive technology. In simple terms, they collect viable healthy semen samples from responsible sperm donors and preserve them according to stipulated international standards. They become the dispensing center of semen to those needy couples or couples referred to them by the physician who treat these patients. Different countries have different rules and regulations depending upon the religion and sociocultural background. Taking one aspect of a complex issue of sperm donation like keeping the anonymity of sperm donor, many countries have different opinions or regulations. Some nations want anonymous sperm donors and in some countries it is suggested that names of sperm donors be made known. In India, sperm donation is common and yet it is a social taboo, rather a social paradox—one does not want to be seen in such clinics; yet many who are desperate to have a child in the family visit these banks. In countries like India, it is said, in desperation, the recipient's father in law (husband's father or brother) comes forward to donate semen samples. What will be the sociological implications to the child born out of such donation will be an ethical issue of great concern. It is said that sperm banks are facilitators receiving semen samples from the donors and giving the samples to the needy. This sounds very pragmatic and unethical. The name sperm bank itself like gene banks dehumanizes human life and dignity. Artificial insemination ("give life and give hope" sounds like "donate blood and save lives") may give hope to desperate parents to have children. Yet, there is lot of difference between saving lives and giving life. Giving life carries social responsibility, which needs to take into account the child's rights.

Author details

Dhastagir Sultan Sheriff[1,2]

1 Reprolabs, Chennai, India

2 Faculty of Medicine, Benghazi University, Benghazi, Libya

*Address all correspondence to: drdsheriff@gmail.com

IntechOpen

References

[1] WHO. 1946. Available from: http://www.who.int/governance/eb/who_constitution_en.pdf/

[2] WHO. 1986. Available from: http://www.who.int/healthpromotion/conferences/previous/ottawa/en/

[3] WHO. 1978. Available from: http://www.who.int/publications/almaata_declaration_en.pdf

[4] Mann S, Stephenson J. Reproductive health and wellbeing—Addressing unmet needs. British Medical Association;BMA. 2018;**20180500**:1-10

[5] Gurunath S, Pandian Z, Richard AR, Bhattacharya S. Defining infertility a systematic review of prevalence studies. Human Reproduction Update. 2011;**17**:575-588

[6] Boivin J, Bunting L, Collins J, Nygren K. International estimates of infertility prevalence and treatment-seeking: Potential need and demand for infertility medical care. Human Reproduction. 2007;**22**:1506-1512

[7] Centers for Disease Control and Prevention. Infertility FAQs; 2013

[8] Kissin DM, Denise JJ, Wanda D. Barfield, monitoring health outcomes of assisted reproductive technology. New England Journal of Medicine. 2014;**371**(1):91-93

[9] Emperaire JC, Ruffié A, Audebert AJ. Ovulation induction by endogenous LH released by the administration of an LHRH agonist after follicular stimulation for in vitro fertilization. Journal de Gynecologie, Obstetrique et Biologie de la Reproduction. 1992;**21**(5):489-494

[10] American Society for Reproductive Medicine. Intrauterine insemination (IU); 2012

[11] Steptoe PC, Edwards RG. Birth after the reimplantation of a human embryo. Lancet. 1978;**2**(8085):366

[12] Asch RH, Ellsworth LR, Balmaceda JP, Wong PC. Pregnancy after translaparoscopic gamete intrafallopian transfer. Lancet. 1984;**2**(8410):1034-1035

[13] De Kretzer D, Dennis P, Hudson B, Leeton J, Lopata A, Outch K, et al. Transfer of a human zygote. Lancet. 1973;**2**(7831):728-729

[14] Verlinsky Y, Ginsberg N, Lifchez A, Valle J, Mo-ise J, Strom CM. Analysis of the first polar body: Preconception genetic diagnosis. Human Reproduction. 1990;**5**(7):826-829

[15] Kamel RM. Assisted reproductive technology after the birth of Louise Brown. Journal of Reproduction and Infertility. 2013;**14**(3):96-109

[16] Son WY, Chung JT, Chian RC, Herrero B, Demirtas E, Elizur S, et al. A 38 h interval between hCG priming and oocyte retrieval increases in vivo and in vitro oocyte maturation rate in programmed IVM cycles. Human Reproduction. 2008;**23**(9):2010-2016

[17] American Society for Reproductive Medicine. Diagnostic evaluation of the infertile female: A committee opinion. Fertility and Sterility. 2015;**103**:e44-e55

[18] Men's Health—Male Factor Infertility. University of Utah Health Sciences Center. 2003. Archived from the Original on 04 July 2007. [Last retrieved on 2007 Nov 11]. Available from: http://web.archive.org/web/20080620064743/http://healthcare.utah.edu/healthinfo/adult/men/infertil.htm

[19] Cooper TG, Noonan E, von Eckardstein S, Auger J, Baker HW,

Behre HM, et al. World Health
Organization reference values for
human semen characteristics. Human
Reproduction Update. 2010;**16**:231-245

[20] Barbieri RL. Yen and Jaffe's
Reproductive Endocrinology
Physiology, Pathophysiology, and
Clinical Management. 8th ed. Canada:
Elsevier; 2018. pp. 556-581

Chapter 2

Medically Assisted Reproduction and the Risk of Adverse Perinatal Outcomes

Jessica Gorgui and Anick Bérard

Abstract

Over 5 million children have been born through *in vitro* fertilization (IVF) across the world. IVF is only one of the many methods of assisted reproduction, which can be used to achieve pregnancy in the context of infertility or subfertility. Since the birth of the first IVF child, Louise Brown, in 1978, a number of researchers have started to study the various impacts of the conception through these methods, on both mothers and children. A growing body of evidence suggests that conception through medically assisted reproduction (MAR) is not without risk. Given that MAR is relatively new and that our look back period is short, there is limited evidence on the risks associated to these procedures, both for the mother and the child. In this chapter, we aim to explore the association between MARs and adverse perinatal outcomes specifically. We will first provide you with an overview of the prevalence and trends of use of these methods around the world, and then delve into the associations between MARs and the risk of perinatal outcomes, namely prematurity, being born with low birth weight and/or small for gestational age, and lastly the impact of MARs on cognitive functions including cerebral palsy, behavioral problems, and autism, which are identified later in the child's life.

Keywords: medically assisted reproduction, prematurity, low birth weight, small for gestational age, delay in cognitive function

1. Introduction

1.1 Infertility and subfertility

Infertility is defined as failure to conceive within 12 months of the first pregnancy attempt [1], while subfertility describes any form or grade of reduced fertility [2, 3].

The National Survey of Family Growth interviewed over 12,000 women of childbearing age (15–44 years old) to estimate the prevalence of infertility in the United States (US) [4]. A woman was considered infertile if she reported she and her partner were continuously cohabiting during the previous 12 months or longer, were sexually active each month, had not used contraception, and had not become pregnant [4]. From 1982 to 2006–2010, the percentage of infertile women based on this definition fell from 8.5 to 6.0% [4]. These estimates are lower than the 12–18% incidence of infertility in the US [5]. The frequency of infertility in nulliparous women (i.e., primary infertility) increased with age and was reported to be: 7.3–9.1% in women 15–34 years old, 25% in the 35–39 year olds, and 30% in the 40–44 year olds [4].

Infertility and subfertility may be due to conditions originating from the male and/or female reproductive systems [6]. Between 8 and 20% of couples will experience difficulty conceiving [6–9]. Between 1982–1985, the World Health Organization (WHO) performed a multicenter study where they attributed 20% of infertility cases to male factors, 38% to female factors, 27% to causal factors identified in both partners, and 15% could not be attributed to either partner [10]. In the following section, we will provide you with an overview of the main causes of infertility.

1.1.1 Male infertility

A cross-sectional survey of men in the United States aged between 15–44 years showed a prevalence of male infertility of 12% [11]. Male infertility accounts for 19–57% of the identified causes of infertility in couples [9]. In about 30–40% of cases of male infertility, the cause remains unknown [11, 12]. Male infertility can be classified into four main categories which we will briefly describe in the following section.

1.1.1.1 Testicular disease: endocrine and systemic disorders

Testicular diseases including *primary testicular defects* account for 30–40% of male infertility [13]. Primary testicular defects can be further classified into: (1) congenital disorders including Klinefelter syndrome [14] and (2) acquired disorders which can be due to infections (e.g., chlamydia) [15] and smoking [16]. *Hypothalamic pituitary diseases* account for 1–2% for male infertility [13]. Secondary hypogonadism can cause gonadotropin deficiencies, which in turn leads to infertility [13]. Secondary hypogonadism can be (1) congenital [17], (2) acquired (e.g., tumors of the pituitary gland [18]) or (3) systemic (e.g., obesity [19]).

1.1.1.2 Genetic disorders of spermatogenesis

Genetic disorders affecting spermatogenesis can be identified in 10–20% of male infertility cases [13]. With the increasing use of genome-wide association studies, genetic disorders have been linked to male infertility [12, 20]. Specifically, microdeletions and substitutions on the Y chromosome are increasingly recognized as genetic causes of azoospermia (i.e., semen without sperm) and severe oligozoospermia (i.e., semen with a sperm concentration < 15 million sperm/mL compared to the norm of >48 million sperm/mL [20]. Additionally, mutations linked to the X chromosome in men have also been linked to azoospermia [21–23].

1.1.1.3 Posttesticular defects

Posttesticular defects lead to disorders of sperm transport, which account for 10–20% of male infertility cases [13]. The epididymis is an important site for sperm maturation and essential to the sperm transport system. The vas deferens transports sperm from the epididymis to the urethra, where they are diluted by secretions from the seminal vesicles and prostate. Abnormalities at any of these sites, particularly the epididymis and vas deferens, can lead to infertility [13]. The causes of these abnormalities include congenital obstructions of the vas deferens and obstruction following an infection (e.g., chlamydia). Additionally, given that sperm must be ejaculated, any disorder of the ejaculatory ducts can also lead to infertility [13].

1.1.1.4 Idiopathic

In 30–40% of male infertility cases, the cause is classified as idiopathic [13]. In these cases, despite attempting to identify potential mechanisms at play, a cause for abnormal sperm number, morphology, or function cannot be identified [13]. Idiopathic causes should be distinguished from unknown causes which is where men with normal semen analysis and no other identified cause for infertility are unable to impregnate an apparently clinically normal female partner.

1.1.2 Female infertility

In terms of female infertility, the main causes of infertility are ovulatory disorders which account for 21–32%, tubal disorders for 14–26%, while endometriosis is responsible in 5–6% of the cases of infertility [6, 9]. Approximately 30% of couples will have both male and female factors contributing to their infertility [6, 9]. When the cause is identified, a treatment plan can be put in place with the physician. The concern however, is that 8–30% of infertility will remain unexplained, which makes the choice of the course of fertility treatment difficult [24]. In the section below, we have provided you with an overview of the main causes attributed to female infertility.

1.1.2.1 Ovaries

1.1.2.1.1 Ovulatory disorders

Infrequent ovulation (oligoovulation) or absent ovulation (anovulation) results in infertility because an oocyte is not available every month for fertilization. WHO classifies ovulatory disorders into three classes [42]:

- Class 1—Hypogonadotropic hypogonadal anovulation occurs in 5–10% of cases. This would describe women with hypothalamic amenorrhea from excessive exercise or low body weight.

- Class 2—Normogonadotropic normoestrogenic anovulation accounts for 70–85% of cases and includes women with polycystic ovary syndrome (PCOS) and hyper/hypothyroidism.

- Class 3—Hypergonadotropic hypoestrogenic anovulation occurs in 10–30% of cases and characterizes women with premature ovarian failure.

1.1.2.1.2 Oocyte aging

Maternal aging is a known factor of female infertility [25]. The decrease in fecundability with aging could be due to a decline in both the quantity and quality of the oocytes [25, 26].

1.1.2.2 Fallopian tubes

Tubal disease and pelvic adhesions prevent normal transport of the oocyte and sperm through the fallopian tube [27]. The primary cause of tubal factor infertility is pelvic inflammatory disease caused by pathogens such as chlamydia or gonorrhea [28]. Tubal and pelvic adhesions could also be a consequence of endometriosis [27].

1.1.2.3 Uterus

Conditions that distort the uterine cavity can result in implantation failure, which may lead to infertility or recurrent pregnancy loss [29]. The most common malformation, a septate uterus, was associated with pregnancy losses >60% and fetal survival rates of 6–28% [30, 31].

1.1.2.4 Endometriosis

Adhesions within the uterus, the fallopian tubes, and/or the pelvic floor caused by endometriosis could be a cause of infertility [27]. This could be mediated through ovulatory dysfunction, defective implantation, alternations within the oocyte, or impaired fertilization among other hypotheses [32].

1.1.2.5 Obesity

Evidence has demonstrated that obese women are at an increased risk of sub-fecundity and infertility [33]. It has been shown that the pathway through which obesity could be a precursor to subfertility/infertility may involve a dysregulation in the hypothalamic-pituitary-ovarian axis as well as decreased oocyte quality and endometrial receptivity [33]. Studies have demonstrated a correlation between higher body mass index (BMI) and poor fertility [33].

1.2. Medically assisted reproduction

Fertility treatments are procedures and/or medication interventions used to initiate a pregnancy. MARs include assisted reproductive techniques (ART) as well as ovarian stimulators (OS). In **Figure 1**, we provide you with a visual classification of MAR techniques as a whole, which we have briefly described below.

1.2.1 Assisted reproductive techniques

ART are defined as procedures that include handling of the oocytes and/or sperm, or embryos to generate a pregnancy [1]. ART methods can be categorized as follows:

1.2.1.1 Intrauterine insemination (IUI)

Intrauterine insemination (IUI) is a procedure in which processed and concentrated motile sperm are placed directly into the uterine cavity, and will often be used when the cause of infertility is related to the male [1].

1.2.1.2 In vitro fertilization (IVF)

In vitro fertilization (IVF) with or without *in vitro* maturation (IVM) is a cycle of procedures in which oocytes are retrieved from ovarian follicles, fertilized *in vitro* then subsequently the resulting embryo(s) are transferred into the uterus [1]. The number of embryos transferred into the uterus largely depends on the common practice imposed by the country where the procedure is performed. A more recent practice is to perform single embryo transfers (SET). This practice was put in place to decrease the odds of producing multiple embryos per pregnancy. However, through the Canadian ART register's (CARTR) last reports in 2012, it was shown

Methods of assisted reproduction

Fertility Medications

ART
Assisted reproductive technology

Ovarian Stimulators

Intrauterine Insemination

In Vitro Fertilisation

Ovulation
Induction

Maturation
and/or release

Embryo
Transfer

ICSI

GIFT/ZIFT

Clomiphene Gonadotropins

GnRH

hCG

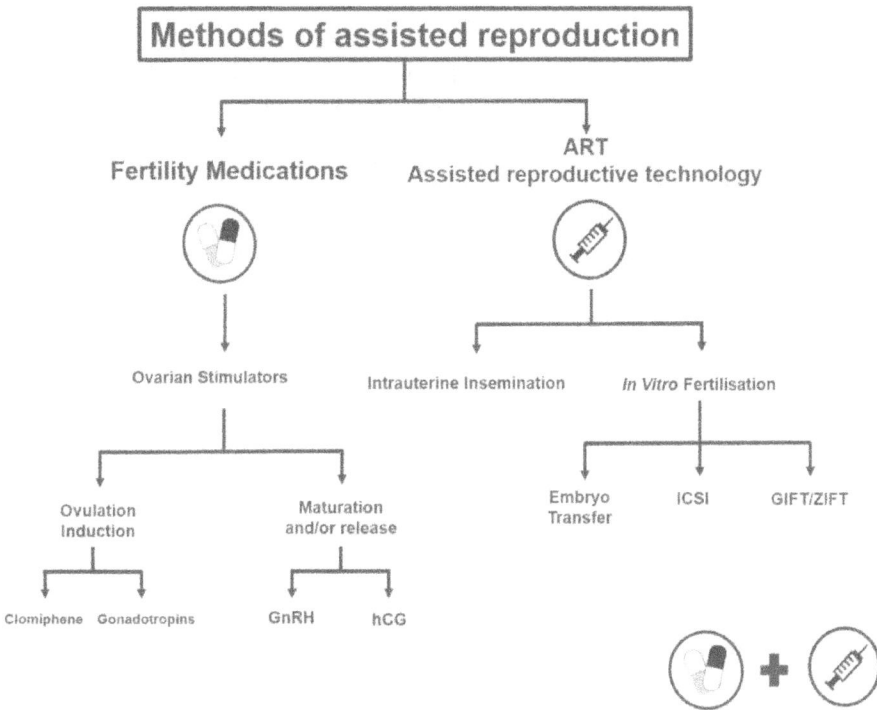

Figure 1.
Overview of the classification of methods of assisted reproduction. Assisted reproductive techniques (ART) are defined as procedures that include handling the oocytes and/or sperm, or embryos to generate a pregnancy (i.e., IVF, ICSI, IUI, in vitro maturation [IVM], assisted hatching [AH], zygote intrafallopian transfer [ZIFT], gamete IFT [GIFT]), while MAR techniques include ART and OS [1]. Depending on the indication of the use of fertility treatments, women will either be given a course of OS, undergo ART procedures alone or will be subjected to a combination of both OS and ART.

that SET has yet to become common practice. Australia/New Zealand and Sweden used SET in >70% of the reported ART cycles involving transfers, compared to 44% in Canada and 14% in Germany [34, 35]. These numbers translated into different rates of multiple pregnancy per country: Australia/New Zealand and Sweden had the lowest rates at 6.9% and 5.9%, respectively, while Canada was at 16.5% and Germany had the highest rates of all reported countries at 32.5% [34, 35]. IVF procedures can be categorized as follows:

- Intra cytoplasmic sperm injection (ICSI) is an *in vitro* procedure in which a single spermatozoon is injected into the oocyte cytoplasm [1].

- Assisted hatching (AH) an *in vitro* procedure in which the zona pellucida of an embryo is either thinned or perforated chemically, mechanically or by laser in order to assist the separation of the blastocyst. The blastocyst is the stage that the embryo reaches 5–6 days following fertilization [1].

- Gamete intrafallopian transfer (GIFT) is an *in vitro* procedure in which both gametes (oocyte and sperm) are transferred into the fallopian tube [1].

- Zygote intrafallopian transfer (ZIFT) is an *in vitro* procedure in which the zygote(s) is/are transferred into the fallopian tube [1].

1.2.2 Ovarian stimulators

Ovarian stimulators (OS) are used to promote the development and ovulation of more than one mature follicle among subfertile women mainly to increase the likelihood of conception [36]. This treatment can be used alone or in combination with IUI, wherein we increase the number of oocytes and sperms together. OS can also be used with other ARTs, described above [1, 37]. In many cases, OS will be used as first line therapy when aiming to treat infertility/subfertility in women or couples. OS alone are more likely to be used in the context of unexplained infertility and age-related subfertility in women [36, 38, 39]. Depending on the underlying cause of infertility, different OS may be used. Mainly, OS can be classified as having two roles as they are either used to induce ovulation (i.e., clomiphene, gonadotropins) or to assist with maturation and/or the release of the oocyte (i.e., human chorionic gonadotropin [hCG], gonadotropin-releasing hormone [GnRH]).

1.2.2.1 Ovulation induction

Infrequent or irregular ovulation (i.e., oligoovulation) unrelated to ovarian failure can usually be treated successfully with ovulation induction (OI); women treated with OI agents achieve fecundability nearly equivalent to that of couples not suffering with infertility or subfertility (i.e., 15–25% probability of achieving a pregnancy in one menstrual cycle) [40]. Agents used for OI tend to be used as a first-line treatment to stimulate the development and ovulation of >1 mature oocyte in women with unexplained or age-related subfertility/infertility [36, 39, 41]. OI agents include clomiphene and gonadotropins. **Clomiphene** is a selective estrogen receptor modulator with both estrogen antagonist and agonist effects that increases gonadotropin release [42]. It is known to be effective in women with normal gonadotropin and estrogen levels but who still have ovulatory dysfunction (WHO Class 2) [42]. **Gonadotropins** are used in women with WHO class 2 who have not been able to ovulate using clomiphene or an insulin sensitizing agent such as metformin (used in women with PCOS). This therapy may also be used in women classified as WHO Class 1 [42].

1.2.2.2 Ovulation maturation and release

Agents used for final ovulation maturation and release are known as trigger shots. The gold standard agent to induce follicular maturation has been hCG which mimics the surge of luteinizing hormone that occurs mid-cycle and allows for the release of the oocyte [43]. GnRH may also be used to replace hCG. Current evidence suggests that GnRH may be used as a first-line treatment in egg donors [43].

2. Trends in medically assisted reproduction use

It has been speculated that fecundability has declined over the years, but results need to be replicated at the scale of large populations in order to be confirmed [44, 45]. Nonetheless, the number of women resorting to fertility treatments remains on the rise. As reported by CARTR, the use of ART has increased steadily over the years, having more than tripled in the last decade [34]. From the participating fertility clinics in the CARTR reports over the years (n = 28–32), 16,315 ART cycles had been performed in 2009 compared to 27,356 cycles in 2012 across Canada [34]. In 2012, Canada had the second lowest number of ART cycles after Sweden (n = 17,628), while the US had the highest number with 176,247 ART cycles performed as reported by the American Society for Reproductive Medicine [34, 35].

Over 5 million children have been born through IVF specifically worldwide [46]. At present, 1–3% of all children in industrialized countries including France, Germany, Italy, Scandinavian countries, and the United States are born through ART [47–49]. Over 1.5 million IVF cycles are performed every year, yielding over 350,000 children annually in Europe, as reported by the European Society of Human Reproduction and Embryology [46].

Between 2010 and 2014, the province of Quebec was the first Canadian province to put in place an assisted reproduction program which provided universal reimbursement for MARs. This program aimed to: (1) reduce multiple pregnancies with the practice of SET, (2) help subfertile/infertile couples to have children, and (3) increase Quebec's birth rate [50]. Following the start of the reimbursement program, reports have shown that MAR represented approximately 2% of all pregnancies [50], of which 43% were from OS without any other ART [51]. Another 20% of women were exposed to OS in combination with IUI, and 33% conceived through IVF [50, 51]. Due to the fact that OS tend to be used the first-line fertility treatment and that it is prescribed with most ARTs, it is the most prevalent exposure [52].

3. Medically assisted reproduction and perinatal outcomes

Since Louise Brown, the first IVF baby, was born in the United Kingdom in 1978, over 5 million children have been born with IVF worldwide [46]. General concerns about the safety of pregnancies resulting from MARs and the health implications of these methods on the resulting child remain, as there is a growing body of evidence supporting the association between these methods and adverse perinatal outcomes [53, 54].

The association between MARs and multiple pregnancies has been studied extensively and is known [51, 55–58]. ART alone and OS use alone have both been associated to increase multiple pregnancies, which occur for two different reasons [57, 59, 60]. On the one hand, ART alone may lead to the transfer of multiple embryos as described above, while on the other hand OS use may lead ovarian hyperstimulation [57, 59–61]. Indeed, ovarian hyperstimulation occurs in more than 40% of stimulated cycles [62]. In the context of ovarian stimulation, it is more difficult to prevent multiple gestations with OS use because it involves the stimulation of ovulation which leads to an unpredictable follicular growth number [61]. As we have described above, the rate of multiple pregnancies associated with ART around the world varies from 5.9 to 32.5% [19, 20]. In a systematic review and meta-analysis performed by Chaabane et al. [63] looking at the association between OS use and multiple pregnancies, they pooled a total of nine studies that had estimates ranging from 1.01 to 50.20 [63]. They calculated a pooled relative risk (RR) of 8.80 with a 95% confidence interval (CI) ranging from 5.09 to 15.20. To put these numbers in context, the rate of multiple pregnancies in the general population is about 3% around the world [64]. These estimates therefore suggest that OS use alone leads to an approximate multiple pregnancy rate of 26% among its' users [46].

ART has also been associated with increased perinatal morbidity and mortality, which the scientific community mainly attributes to the increased risk of multiple births, the use of these technologies themselves, as well as the underlying condition for which these methods are used, which is the infertility factor [54, 65–70]. In fact, it is generally well accepted that multiple pregnancies occurring in the context of fertility treatments due to the transfer of multiple embryos are associated with being born premature (<37 weeks of gestation) or at a low birth weight (LBW;

<2500 g at birth) [71]. These complications, among others, carry long-term impacts on the child, which we will explore throughout this chapter.

Researchers have been making an effort to evaluate adverse risks associated with MARs in singleton babies specifically. In fact, MAR-conceived singletons have been shown to be at increased risk of very preterm (28 to <32 gestational weeks) and moderately preterm birth (32 to <37 gestational weeks), LBW, small for gestational age (SGA; weight below the 10th percentile for their gestational age), neonatal intensive care unit (ICU) admissions (odds ratio [OR], 1.27; 95%CI, 1.16–1.40), and overall perinatal mortality (OR, 1.68; 95%CI, 1.11–2.55) compared to spontaneously conceived singletons [72, 73]. In line with these findings, IVF-conceived children tend to be hospitalized for longer (n = 9.5 days versus 3.6 days in non-IVF children), and use more in-patient care than their non-IVF counterparts in the neonatal period and later in life due to increased risk of asthma, cerebral palsy, congenital malformations, and infections [74]. It could be speculated that these results are due to prematurity or multiplicity, but this observation persisted when restricted to term infants and singletons, respectively [74].

A growing body of evidence suggests that children conceived through ART are phenotypically and biochemically different from naturally conceived children [75]. Indeed, MAR involves hyperstimulation, manipulation, and culture of gametes/ embryos at the most vulnerable stage of development [76, 77]. ART has been implied to affect the epigenetic control in early embryogenesis [78, 79]. In fact, MARs have been associated with an increased risk of imprinting disorders both in experimental and epidemiological studies [80, 81]. Furthermore, we must take into consideration the impact of iatrogenic factors including gamete manipulations and ovulation hyperstimulation, as well as the initial underlying cause of infertility as discussed above.

In the following section of the chapter, we will present the associations between MARs and the risks of the main perinatal outcomes (i.e., prematurity, LBW, SGA) as well as long-term cognitive outcomes.

3.1 Prematurity

In the previous section, we discussed the known association between MARs and the risk of multiplicity. Multiplicity has been shown to increase the risk of preterm birth by 6-fold [82]. More recently, efforts have been made by the scientific community to evaluate the contribution of MARs on the risk of prematurity among singletons specifically. As such, we are able to tease out the role of multiplicity in the association between the MARs themselves and the risk of prematurity [83, 84].

Evidence from a systematic review of matched controlled studies showed that MAR-conceived singletons were at an increased risk for very preterm (28 to <32 weeks' gestation) and moderately preterm birth (32 to <37 weeks' gestation), compared to spontaneously conceived singletons [72, 73]. The RRs reported for 13 studies ranged from 0.57 (0.21–1.56) performed among 118 women [85] to 8.00 (1.87–34.2) performed among 240 women [86]. The general consensus among these 13 matched studies was that the risk of preterm birth was doubled [72]. Most studies included in this systematic review adjusted for maternal age and parity by design (i.e., matched case-control studies), but most failed to perform adjustments for confounding variables such as smoking, socio-economic status, and pre-existing chronic conditions [72]. Further supporting these results, ART users were 3.27 times more at risk of prematurity than non-ART users (RR, 3.27; 95%CI, 2.03–5.28). ART was also associated with a doubling of the risk of delivering moderately preterm (RR, 2.05; 95%CI, 1.71–2.47) [87–89]. To put these results in context, the prevalence of prematurity is of 7.8% in Canada and 10% in the USA [90]. These results indicate that among MAR-conceived children, the prevalence of prematurity could be estimated at 15% or higher.

We found that the current literature does not appropriately take into account the different fertility treatments separately and do not create the necessary distinction between OS and ART [72, 87–89]. MARs are either pooled all together or only IVF or ICSI are considered in analyses. Further studies are required to explore the biological mechanisms through which these methods could cause premature birth/delivery, which will only be possible once we have assessed each MAR distinctively.

3.2 Low birth weight

ART conceptions have been associated with being born LBW. Results have mainly been attributed to higher rates of multiple pregnancies and prematurity among MAR conceptions [91]. Recent meta-analyses have shown that the higher rates of LBW are observed in both IVF singletons as well as twins, respectively, compared to natural conceptions [92, 93]. When comparing singleton ART-conceived children to those who were spontaneously conceived, we observed a 1.70-fold increase in the risk of LBW among ART singletons (RR, 1.70; 95%CI, 1.50–1.92) [72]. In Canada, the prevalence of LBW was of 6.2% in 2013 [94] which is lower than the prevalence reported in the USA in 2016, which was of approximately 8% [95]. To put these numbers into context, this would mean that among ART-conceived children, the prevalence of LBW would be between 11 and 13%. Additionally, when comparing singletons conceived through ART to those who were naturally conceived, the meta-analysis showed a 3-fold increase in the risk of being born very LBW which is defined as a birth weight of <1500 g (RR, 3.00; 95%CI, 2.07–4.36) [72].

A number of studies have shown that IVF-conceived singletons were at an increased risk of being born LBW, even following adjustment for gestational age which is a known confounder [96–102], while two large prospective studies and one matched case-control did not observe any differences following adjustments [85, 103, 104]. Through they did not all adjust for the same variables, the two prospective studies took into account maternal age, gestational age, education, marital status, BMI, intrauterine exposure to smoking/alcohol/coffee as well as the sex of the child, parity, and time since last pregnancy [103, 104].

Aside from the body of evidence examining the association between ART and LBW, the exposure to OS has also been associated with LBW when compared with spontaneous conceptions in conceptions with [68, 105, 106] and without IVF [101, 107].

It has been hypothesized in this context that an alteration in oocyte quality, decreased receptivity of the endometrium or the production of a poor implantation environment may play a role in this observation [101, 107]. These could in part be mediated through the increased levels of estradiol which could impair the implantation process and this hypothesis has been confirmed in animal studies [91].

3.3 Small for gestational age

In the context of infertility treatments, we have discussed the negative implications of OS on the uterine environment. As such, oocyte manipulation as well as hormonal triggers during implantation could be key players in the mother's response to growth factors [107]. In fact, the capacity of the placental system to transfer nutrients to the fetus as well as the condition of the maternal endocrine system will determine, along with genetics, whether or not the fetus will follow an expectedly normal growth curve during the gestational period [108]. Being born SGA describes newborns who are smaller than the norm for their gestational age established by the average growth curve [109]. It is important to note that definitions of SGA are population-dependent as growth curves differ from one country to another [109].

Limited evidence exists on the association between MARs and SGA. However, when comparing singleton IVF-conceived children to those who were spontaneously conceived, studies observed a 1.4–1.6 fold increase in the risk of SGA among IVF singletons [72, 110, 111]. An additional study published by the United Kingdom government looked at this association and found a significant increased risk of SGA when comparing IVF to spontaneous conception (RR, 1.98; 95%CI, 1.21–3.24) and also when comparing OS use alone to spontaneous conception (RR, 1.71; 95%CI, 1.09–2.69) [112]. In low- to middle income countries, the prevalence of SGA births is of approximately 27% while in industrialized countries, the prevalence ranges around 5–10% [113]. Based on these prevalences, this would indicate that prevalences of SGA among IVF-conceived children could range from 8.5–45%.

Current evidence is suggestive of an association between MARs and conceiving babies that are SGA. Mechanisms leading to growth restriction *in utero* are those discussed above when describing the probable etiology for the increased risk of LBW [91]. Additional large-scale epidemiological studies are required to confirm these results, as well as to generate further hypotheses to be tested in mechanistic animal studies.

3.4 Long-term cognitive outcomes

Environmental factors that come into play in the early stages of embryonic development can interact with the genotype and alter the capacity of the organism to cope with this environment later in life, therefore modulating a child's susceptibility to disease [114, 115]. Evidence suggests that MAR-conceived children are phenotypically and biochemically different from the spontaneously conceived [75]. MAR involves hyperstimulation, manipulation, and culture of gametes/embryos at the most vulnerable stage of development [76, 77]. However, increased risk of neurodevelopmental disorders in MAR-conceived children may be unrelated to the procedure/treatment itself; MAR has been associated with increased risk of multiple gestation [63], which in turn increases the risk of PTB, LBW, and SGA newborns as we have described in detail in previous sections of the chapter [104, 111, 116]. These adverse outcomes are strongly associated with a range of long-term child outcomes, including vision impairment, cerebral palsy (CP), and neurodevelopmental deficits [46, 117–120]. With the current state of the evidence, results support the hypothesis that MARs could be a contributing factor to the recent increase in the prevalence of neurodevelopmental disorders.

3.4.1 Cerebral palsy

CP is the most common motor disability in childhood. Approximately 1 in 323 children (0.3%) has been identified with CP according to estimates from CDC's Autism and Developmental Disabilities Monitoring Network. Population-based studies worldwide report prevalence estimates of CP ranging from 1.5 to more than 4 per 1000 live births or children of a defined age range [121–124].

Very few groups have evaluated the association between MARs and CP. Most available results stem from studies performed within large registries available in the Scandinavian countries, namely Denmark, Finland, and Sweden. In 2009,

Hvidtjørn et al. performed a systematic review and meta-analysis to provide an overview of the results pertaining to this association [125]. A total of nine studies were included in this review [74, 126–133]. They were conscious to separate results by parity (e.g., all children combined, singletons, twins, and triplets) and to isolate estimates that had been adjusted for PTD, as it is a known risk factor for CP [125]. The outcome was defined by appropriate diagnostic codes of the *International Statistical Classification of Diseases, 10th Revision (ICD-10)*. Only two studies used records from rehabilitations centers, one from questionnaires which were later confirmed by discharge registers. All other studies obtained their information on CP diagnoses from hospital discharge registers.

Among studies looking at all children combined, adjusted ORs ranged between 0.88 and 3.7 [74, 126, 127, 129, 132]. The strongest reported association was that of Strömberg et al. with a significant 3.7-fold increased CP risk when comparing IVF to non-IVF children [132]. After adjusting for PTD, the point estimate was reduced to 2.9 but remained significant [132]. Other studies found no significant association when they adjusted for PTD. Among singleton studies, the tendency was towards an increased CP risk among IVF singletons when compared to their non-IVF counterparts [126–128, 132]. The results of the meta-analysis showed an overall significant 1.8-fold increase (OR, 1.82; 95%CI, [1.31–2.52]) in CP when comparing IVF singletons to non-IVF singletons [125].

Among studies including twins and triplets, the ORs were variable and ranged from 0.6 and 1.5, and most results were not significant [126, 127, 130–133]. Despite their large sample sizes, they had a low number of MAR-conceived children with CP, with numbers ranging from 3 to 15. Additionally, studies did not take into account PTD which could potentially be biasing these results [126, 127, 130–133].

Overall, this systematic review of the literature and meta-analysis suggests that there is evidence supporting the implication of MARs, specifically IVF, in the increased risk of CP. To put these results in context, CP remains a rare outcome with a prevalence of 0.3% on average. These results would suggest that among MAR-conceived children, the prevalence of CP could range between 0.6% and 1%. The increased risk of CP among IVF-born children could be in part explained by the known association between IVF and PTD [125]. Indeed, a more recent study published in 2012 indicates that among MAR-conceived children, the risk of neurodevelopmental outcomes, including CP, is more pronounced among those that are born extremely preterm (22–26 weeks' gestation) [134].

3.4.2 Autism

As discussed above, ART-conceived children are phenotypically and biochemically different from naturally conceived children, likely due to the manipulation of gametes and embryos at such a vulnerable stage of development [75–77]. MARs have been associated with an increased risk of imprinting disorders, which in turn can lead to ASD [80, 81]. Studies have shown that ASD risk is 1.5 to 2 times higher among MAR-conceived children compared with their spontaneously conceived counterparts [125, 135–138]. However, these associations were reduced after adjustments for sociodemographic and perinatal variables including multiplicity, PTD, SGA, maternal diabetes, hypertension and preeclampsia, and cesarean deliver. One small case-control study (n = 942) performed in India looked at the association between exposure to OS and the risk of ASD (measured through questionnaires), and identified a 2-fold increased risk of ASD when compared to their spontaneously-conceived counterparts [139]. To put these results in context, the estimated prevalence of ASD has increased over time from 0.05% in the 1960s [140] to 1.46% today in the USA [141] and is reported to be 1.36% in Quebec,

Canada [142]. This would indicate that among IVF-conceived children, the prevalence of ASD could be of approximately 2%.

On the contrary, other groups have yielded reassuring results when considering ASD as an outcome [143, 144]. Overall, findings remain inconsistent as risk estimate ranges are wide and variable across studies [145]. It is important to note that a number of differences among these studies have been identified, and could therefore explain the disparity among results. Specifically, studies were performed in small populations, which makes it especially difficult to study a rare outcome such as ASD [125, 139, 145]. Additionally, ASD definitions were variable across studies, and were often non-specific which could be due to differences in diagnostic criteria. Some studies used questionnaires which are subject to recall bias, while other studies used diagnostic codes through a registry. However, it is also important to note that over the years, diagnostic criteria used to define ASD have changed between versions of the *Diagnostic and Statistical Manual of Mental Disorders* (4th versus 5th editions) [146, 147]. Lastly, we have identified that there is a lack of evidence and consideration of the immediate and long-term effect of OS alone as most studies focused on IVF or MARs in general without including the pharmacological approach [125, 145].

Throughout this chapter, we have seen that MARs increase the risk of multiple gestation, prematurity, being born with LBW, and SGA. As such, the observed increased risk of ASD in MAR-conceived children may be due to reasons unrelated to the procedure or treatment itself. As we know, MAR has been associated with increased risk for multiple gestations [63], which in turn increase the risk for prematurity, LBW, and SGA babies [104, 111, 116]. We know that these are major risk factors for neurodevelopmental deficits, including ASD [46, 117]. The main question that remains is how MAR techniques contribute to the increased ASD risk. The identified limitations as well as the inconsistency of results underline the importance to produce more evidence on this association by including all exposures to MARs as identified through this chapter.

3.4.3 Behavioral problems

Most studies presented herein measured behavioral problems through a questionnaire which included a Strengths and Difficulties Questionnaire (SDQ). The SDQ is a validated tool comprised of 25 items which aims to assess the psychological adjustment of children and youths [148]. Based on this questionnaire, behavioral problems were defined as having emotional symptoms, hyperactivity, conduct problems, prosocial behavior, and problems with their peers [148]. Depending on the study group, the mother, the teacher or the child themselves (i.e., later as an adult) had filled out the questionnaire to assess the outcome.

The rationale for the evaluation of this association is that couples who undergo a long waiting time before being able to conceive and/or who have had to undergo lengthy fertility treatments tend to experience significant amounts of stress and anxiety during the process. Studies have shown that this increased period of stress may affect their ability to adapt to their new parenting role, which in consequence may influence their children's behavioral and emotional development [149–151]. Animal studies suggest that this response may be largely due to the activity of the stress-responsive hypothalamic-pituitary-adrenal axis and its end-product, which is cortisol [151]. Higher levels of cortisol in the mother during the pregnancy are translated into higher levels in the offspring, which in turn can influence the child's behavior [151]. Further supporting this theory, studies found that women who suffered with symptoms of anxiety late in their pregnancy (32+ weeks' gestation) had higher levels of cortisol in their blood following adjustments for sociodemographic status, gestational age, parity, and lifestyle factors (i.e., smoking and alcohol consumption) [152, 153].

At both 5 and 7 years of age, the mean behavioral difficulties score was significantly higher in the ART-children when compared to children born through spontaneous conception, even after adjusting for other confounding variables [154]. Indeed, a study performed in the Millenium Cohort comprised of 18,552 women, ART-conceived children had double the risk of having children with peer problems at 5 years of age (OR, 2.56; 95%CI, 1.14–5.77—model adjusted for maternal age, age of the child, sex of the child, household socioeconomic status, family type, maternal qualifications) [154]. A weaker association was observed at age 7 and was non-significant. It was also shown that at the age of 5, ART-conceived children seem to have increased emotional difficulties when compared to those who were spontaneously conceived (adjusted OR, 1.80; 95%CI, 0.86, 3.79). Additionally at age 7, increased peer problems remained (adjusted OR, 1.90; 95%CI, 0.90, 3.98) [154]. Studies have shown that children conceived spontaneously, whether or not mothers/couples struggled with infertility, had similar behavioral patterns [155–159]. These results therefore suggest that the underlying cause of infertility in the parents is unlikely related to resulting behavioral patters in children [159].

To put these results in context, it is estimated that 1 in 10 individuals (10%) will suffer with behavioral problems throughout their life [160]. These results suggest that among MAR-conceived children, the prevalence of behavioral problems could be estimated at 20%.

On the contrary, other studies performed among ART-conceived children did not exhibit any more behavioral problems than their naturally conceived counterparts [125, 155–158]. Some of these studies, unlike the others we have presented, even suggested a more positive relationship between parents and ART-conceived children [159, 161, 162]. Contrary to the previous theory about higher levels of stress among these parents, these results are explained by the fact that ART-conceived children may have a higher desirability factor than their spontaneously conceived counterparts (i.e., planned and unplanned) [159].

Despite the differences in observed results, there seems to be a trend towards an implication of MARs in the development of behavioral problems later in life. The current evidence on behavioral problems suggests that there is a need for the development of long-term surveillance programs (i.e., registries and databases) for MAR-conceived children as of the age of 5 and until early adulthood.

4. Conclusions

The prevalence of MAR use around the world has been increased over the last years. With a noticeable surge of infertility/subfertility among women of childbearing age, these numbers are expected to remain on the rise. Through this chapter, we evaluated the current state of the literature and showed that MARs have been associated with a number of significant adverse perinatal outcomes, which have repercussions on the child later in life, but also on their parents, and society. MAR-conceived children seem to have poorer health overall with increased healthcare utilization largely due to an increased prevalence of prematurity, being born LBW or SGA, and later in life, being more at risk for behavioral problems, cerebral palsy, and autism among other neurodevelopmental outcomes. Decision makers as well as healthcare professionals should be aware of the repercussions that these methods could have on the mother as well as the child, and appropriately inform mothers and couples seeking these therapies to achieve pregnancy in the context of infertility. Further stufies are needed to present more evidence to strenghten the findings related to perinatal outcomes when conceiving through MARs.

Acknowledgements

Dr. Bérard is the recipient of a career award from the Fonds de la Recherche en Santé du Québec (FRQS) and is on the endowment Research Chair of the Famille Louis-Boivin, which funds research on Medications, Pregnancy, and Lactation at the Faculty of Pharmacy of the University of Montreal. Jessica Gorgui is the recipient of the Sainte-Justine Hospital Foundation/Foundation of the Stars doctoral scholarship as well as the FRQS doctoral award.

Conflict of interest

JG and AB have no conflicts of interest to report.

Author details

Jessica Gorgui[1,2] and Anick Bérard[1,2]*

1 Research Center, CHU Sainte-Justine, Montreal, Quebec, Canada

2 Faculty of Pharmacy, University of Montreal, Montreal, Quebec, Canada

*Address all correspondence to: anick.berard@umontreal.ca

IntechOpen

References

[1] Zegers-Hochschild F et al. International Committee for Monitoring Assisted Reproductive Technology (ICMART) and the World Health Organization (WHO) revised glossary of ART terminology, 2009. Fertility and Sterility. 2009;**92**(5):1520-1524

[2] Gnoth C et al. Definition and prevalence of subfertility and infertility. Human Reproduction. 2005;**20**(5): 1144-1147

[3] Jenkins J et al. European classification of infertility taskforce (ECIT) response to Habbema et al., 'Towards less confusing terminology in reproductive medicine: A proposal'. Human Reproduction. 2004;**19**(12):2687-2688

[4] Chandra A, Copen CE, Stephen EH. Infertility and impaired fecundity in the United States, 1982–2010: Data from the National Survey of Family Growth. National Health Statistics Reports (NHSR). 2013;(67):1-18

[5] Thoma ME et al. Prevalence of infertility in the United States as estimated by the current duration approach and a traditional constructed approach. Fertility and Sterility. 2013; **99**(5):1324-1331.e1

[6] Hull MG et al. Population study of causes, treatment, and outcome of infertility. British Medical Journal (Clinical Research Ed.). 1985;**291**(6510): 1693-1697

[7] Case AM. Infertility evaluation and management. Strategies for family physicians. Canadian Family Physician. 2003;**49**:1465-1472

[8] Oakley L, Doyle P, Maconochie N. Lifetime prevalence of infertility and infertility treatment in the UK: Results from a population-based survey of

reproduction. Human Reproduction. 2008;**23**(2):447-450

[9] Thonneau P et al. Incidence and main causes of infertility in a resident population (1,850,000) of three French regions (1988–1989). Human Reproduction. 1991;**6**(6):811-816

[10] World Health Organisation. Towards more objectivity in diagnosis and management of male infertility. Results of a world health organization multicenter study. International Journal of Andrology. 1987;7:1-53

[11] Louis JF et al. The prevalence of couple infertility in the United States from a male perspective: Evidence from a nationally representative sample. Andrology. 2013;**1**(5):741-748

[12] Krausz C, Chianese C. Genetic testing and counselling for male infertility. Current Opinion in Endocrinology, Diabetes, and Obesity. 2014;**21**(3):244-250

[13] de Kretser DM. Male infertility. Lancet. 1997;**349**(9054):787-790

[14] McLachlan RI, O'Bryan MK. Clinical review#: State of the art for genetic testing of infertile men. The Journal of Clinical Endocrinology and Metabolism. 2010;**95**(3):1013-1024

[15] Umapathy E. STD/HIV association: Effects on semen characteristics. Archives of Andrology. 2005;**51**(5): 361-365

[16] Vine MF et al. Cigarette smoking and sperm density: A meta-analysis. Fertility and Sterility. 1994;**61**(1):35-43

[17] Spratt DI et al. The spectrum of abnormal patterns of gonadotropin-releasing hormone secretion in men with idiopathic hypogonadotropic

hypogonadism: Clinical and laboratory correlations. The Journal of Clinical Endocrinology and Metabolism. 1987; **64**(2):283-291

[18] Freeman DA. Steroid hormone-producing tumors of the adrenal, ovary, and testes. Endocrinology and Metabolism Clinics of North America. 1991;**20**(4):751-766

[19] Isidori AM et al. Leptin and androgens in male obesity: Evidence for leptin contribution to reduced androgen levels. The Journal of Clinical Endocrinology and Metabolism. 1999; **84**(10):3673-3680

[20] Ferlin A et al. Molecular and clinical characterization of Y chromosome microdeletions in infertile men: A 10-year experience in Italy. The Journal of Clinical Endocrinology and Metabolism. 2007;**92**(3):762-770

[21] Teng YN et al. Association of a single-nucleotide polymorphism of the deleted-in-azoospermia-like gene with susceptibility to spermatogenic failure. The Journal of Clinical Endocrinology and Metabolism. 2002;**87**(11): 5258-5264

[22] Yatsenko AN et al. X-linked TEX11 mutations, meiotic arrest, and azoospermia in infertile men. The New England Journal of Medicine. 2015; **372**(22):2097-2107

[23] Zou S et al. Association study between polymorphisms of PRMT6, PEX10, SOX5, and nonobstructive azoospermia in the Han Chinese population. Biology of Reproduction. 2014;**90**(5):96

[24] ESHRE. Capri Workshop. Infertility revisited: The state of the art today and tomorrow. European Society for Human Reproduction and Embryology. Human Reproduction. 1996;**11**(8):1779-1807

[25] Crawford NM, Steiner AZ. Age-related infertility. Obstetrics and Gynecology Clinics of North America. 2015;**42**(1):15-25

[26] Sauer MV. Reproduction at an advanced maternal age and maternal health. Fertility and Sterility. 2015; **103**(5):1136-1143

[27] Abrao MS, Muzii L, Marana R. Anatomical causes of female infertility and their management. International Journal of Gynaecology and Obstetrics. 2013;**123**(Supp. 2):S18-S24

[28] Haggerty CL et al. Risk of sequelae after chlamydia trachomatis genital infection in women. The Journal of Infectious Diseases. 2010;**201** (Supplement_2):S134-S155

[29] Steinkeler JA et al. Female infertility: A systematic approach to radiologic imaging and diagnosis. Radiographics. 2009;**29**(5):1353-1370

[30] Homer HA, Li T-C, Cooke ID. The septate uterus: A review of management and reproductive outcome. Fertility and Sterility. 2000;**73**(1):1-14

[31] Grimbizis GF et al. Clinical implications of uterine malformations and hysteroscopic treatment results. Human Reproduction Update. 2001; **7**(2):161-174

[32] Halis G, Arici A. Endometriosis and inflammation in infertility. Annals of the New York Academy of Sciences. 2004;**1034**(1):300-315

[33] Talmor A, Dunphy B. Female obesity and infertility. Best Practice & Research Clinical Obstetrics & Gynaecology. 2015;**29**(4):498-506

[34] Gunby J. Assisted Reproductive Technologies (ART) in Canada: 2011 Results from the Canadian ART Register (CARTR). 2011. Available from: https://

www.cfas.ca/images/stories/pdf/
CARTR_2011_v4.pdf

[35] Centers for Disease Control and
Prevention, American Society for
Reproductive Medicine, Society for
Assisted Reproductive Technology. 2012
Assisted Reproductive Technology
National Summary. 2012. Available
from: http://nccd.cdc.gov/DRH_ART/
Apps/NationalSummaryReport.aspx

[36] Practice Committee of the American
Society for Reproductive Medicine.
Multiple gestation associated with
infertility therapy: An American Society
for Reproductive Medicine practice
committee opinion. Fertility and
Sterility. 2012;**97**(4):825-834

[37] Fauser BC, Devroey P, Macklon NS.
Multiple birth resulting from ovarian
stimulation for subfertility treatment.
Lancet. 2005;**365**(9473):1807-1816

[38] Guzick DS et al. Efficacy of
superovulation and intrauterine
insemination in the treatment of
infertility. National Cooperative
Reproductive Medicine Network. The
New England Journal of Medicine. 1999;
340(3):177-183

[39] Barrington KJ, Janvier A. The
paediatric consequences of assisted
reproductive technologies, with special
emphasis on multiple pregnancies. Acta
Paediatrica. 2013;**102**(4):340-348

[40] Collins JA et al. Treatment-
independent pregnancy among infertile
couples. The New England Journal of
Medicine. 1983;**309**(20):1201-1206

[41] Stovall DW, Guzick DS. Current
management of unexplained infertility.
Current Opinion in Obstetrics &
Gynecology. 1993;**5**(2):228-233

[42] Pacchiarotti A et al. Ovarian
stimulation protocol in IVF: An up-
to-date review of the literature. Current

Pharmaceutical Biotechnology. 2016;
17(4):303-315

[43] Castillo JC et al. Pharmaceutical
Options for Triggering of Final Oocyte
Maturation in ART. Vol. 2014. 2014. p. 7

[44] Olsen J, Zhu JL, Ramlau-Hansen
CH. Has fertility declined in recent
decades? Acta Obstetricia et
Gynecologica Scandinavica. 2011;**90**(2):
129-135

[45] Sallmen M et al. Has human fertility
declined over time? Why we may never
know. Epidemiology. 2005;**16**(4):
494-499

[46] Bauquis C. The world's Number of
IVF and ICSI Babies Has Now Reached a
Calculated Total of 5 Million. Brussels:
ESHRE; 2012

[47] Andersen AN et al. Assisted
reproductive technology in Europe,
2003. Results generated from European
registers by ESHRE. Human
Reproduction. 2007;**22**(6):1513-1525

[48] Juul S, Karmaus W, Olsen J.
Regional differences in waiting time to
pregnancy: Pregnancy-based surveys
from Denmark, France, Germany, Italy
and Sweden. The European Infertility
and Subfecundity Study Group. Human
Reproduction. 1999;**14**(5):1250-1254

[49] Wright VC et al. Assisted
reproductive technology surveillance—
United States, 2005. MMWR
Surveillance Summaries. 2008;**57**(5):
1-23

[50] Salois R. Summary Advisory on
Assisted Reproduction in Quebec—
Report by the Commissaire à la santé et
au Bien-être du Québec. 2014

[51] Chaabane S et al. Ovarian
stimulators, intrauterine insemination,
and assisted reproductive technologies
use and the risk of major congenital

malformations—The AtRISK Study. Birth Defects Research. Part B, Developmental and Reproductive Toxicology. 2016;**107**(3):136-147

[52] Berard A, Sheehy O. The Quebec Pregnancy Cohort—Prevalence of medication use during gestation and pregnancy outcomes. PLoS One. 2014; **9**(4):e93870

[53] Schieve LA et al. Are children born after assisted reproductive technology at increased risk for adverse health outcomes? Obstetrics and Gynecology. 2004;**103**(6):1154-1163

[54] Sutcliffe AG, Ludwig M. Outcome of assisted reproduction. Lancet. 2007; **370**(9584):351-359

[55] Farhi A et al. Maternal and neonatal health outcomes following assisted reproduction. Reproductive Biomedicine Online. 2013;**26**(5): 454-461

[56] Schieve LA. Multiple-gestation pregnancies after assisted reproductive technology treatment: Population trends and future directions. Womens Health (Lond). 2007;**3**(3):301-307

[57] Chaabane S et al. Association between ovarian stimulators with or without intrauterine insemination, and assisted reproductive technologies on multiple births. American Journal of Obstetrics and Gynecology. 2015; **213**(4):511 e1-511 e14

[58] Zhu JL et al. Infertility, infertility treatment and twinning: The Danish National Birth Cohort. Human Reproduction. 2007;**22**(4):1086-1090

[59] Kallen B, Olausson PO, Nygren KG. Neonatal outcome in pregnancies from ovarian stimulation. Obstetrics and Gynecology. 2002;**100**(3):414-419

[60] Zhu L et al. Maternal and live-birth outcomes of pregnancies following

assisted reproductive technology: A retrospective cohort study. Scientific Reports. 2016;**6**:35141

[61] Baerwald AR, Adams GP, Pierson RA. Ovarian antral folliculogenesis during the human menstrual cycle: A review. Human Reproduction Update. 2012;**18**(1):73-91

[62] Gleicher N et al. Reducing the risk of high-order multiple pregnancy after ovarian stimulation with gonadotropins. The New England Journal of Medicine. 2000;**343**(1):2-7

[63] Chaabane S et al. Ovarian stimulation, intrauterine insemination, multiple pregnancy and major congenital malformations: A systematic review and Meta-analysis—The ART_ Rev Study. Current Drug Safety. 2016; **11**(3):222-261

[64] Collins J. Global epidemiology of multiple birth. Reproductive Biomedicine Online. 2007;**15**(Supp. 3): 45-52

[65] Allen C et al. Pregnancy and perinatal outcomes after assisted reproduction: A comparative study. Irish Journal of Medical Science. 2008; **177**(3):233-241

[66] Allen VM, Wilson RD, Cheung A. Pregnancy outcomes after assisted reproductive technology. Journal of Obstetrics and Gynaecology Canada. 2006;**28**(3):220-233

[67] Basatemur E, Sutcliffe A. Follow-up of children born after ART. Placenta. 2008;**29 Suppl B**:135-140

[68] Chung K et al. Factors influencing adverse perinatal outcomes in pregnancies achieved through use of in vitro fertilization. Fertility and Sterility. 2006;**86**(6):1634-1641

[69] Ludwig AK et al. Post-neonatal health and development of children

born after assisted reproduction: A systematic review of controlled studies. European Journal of Obstetrics, Gynecology, and Reproductive Biology. 2006;**127**(1):3-25

[70] Wisborg K, Ingerslev HJ, Henriksen TB. IVF and stillbirth: A prospective follow-up study. Human Reproduction. 2010;**25**(5):1312-1316

[71] Hart R, Norman RJ. The longer-term health outcomes for children born as a result of IVF treatment: Part I—General health outcomes. Human Reproduction Update. 2013;**19**(3):232-243

[72] Helmerhorst FM et al. Perinatal outcome of singletons and twins after assisted conception: A systematic review of controlled studies. BMJ. 2004; **328**(7434):261

[73] Thomson F et al. Obstetric outcome in women with subfertility. BJOG: An International Journal of Obstetrics and Gynaecology. 2005;**112**(5):632-637

[74] Ericson A et al. Hospital care utilization of infants born after IVF. Human Reproduction. 2002;**17**(4): 929-932

[75] Savage T et al. Childhood outcomes of assisted reproductive technology. Human Reproduction. 2011;**26**(9): 2392-2400

[76] Fleming TP et al. The embryo and its future. Biology of Reproduction. 2004;**71**(4):1046-1054

[77] Young LE. Imprinting of genes and the Barker hypothesis. Twin Research. 2001;**4**(5):307-317

[78] Gomes MV et al. Abnormal methylation at the KvDMR1 imprinting control region in clinically normal children conceived by assisted reproductive technologies. Molecular Human Reproduction. 2009;**15**(8): 471-477

[79] Katari S et al. DNA methylation and gene expression differences in children conceived in vitro or in vivo. Human Molecular Genetics. 2009;**18**(20): 3769-3778

[80] Horsthemke B, Ludwig M. Assisted reproduction: The epigenetic perspective. Human Reproduction Update. 2005;**11**(5):473-482

[81] van Montfoort AP et al. Assisted reproduction treatment and epigenetic inheritance. Human Reproduction Update. 2012;**18**(2):171-197

[82] Blondel B et al. The impact of the increasing number of multiple births on the rates of preterm birth and low birthweight: An international study. American Journal of Public Health. 2002;**92**(8):1323-1330

[83] Chambers GM et al. Hospital utilization, costs and mortality rates during the first 5 years of life: A population study of ART and non-ART singletons. Human Reproduction. 2014; **29**(3):601-610

[84] Chambers GM et al. Hospital costs of multiple-birth and singleton-birth children during the first 5 years of life and the role of assisted reproductive technology. JAMA Pediatrics. 2014; **168**(11):1045-1053

[85] Isaksson R, Gissler M, Tiitinen A. Obstetric outcome among women with unexplained infertility after IVF: A matched case-control study. Human Reproduction. 2002;**17**(7):1755-1761

[86] Verlaenen H et al. Singleton pregnancy after in vitro fertilization: Expectations and outcome. Obstetrics and Gynecology. 1995;**86**(6):906-910

[87] Koivurova S et al. Neonatal outcome and congenital malformations in children born after in-vitro fertilization. Human Reproduction. 2002;**17**(5): 1391-1398

[88] Dhont M et al. Perinatal outcome of pregnancies after assisted reproduction: A case-control study. American Journal of Obstetrics and Gynecology. 1999; **181**(3):688-695

[89] Dhont M et al. Perinatal outcome of pregnancies after assisted reproduction: A case-control study. Journal of Assisted Reproduction and Genetics. 1997; **14**(10):575-580

[90] Blencowe H et al. Born too soon: The global epidemiology of 15 million preterm births. Reproductive Health. 2013;**10 Supp. 1**:S2

[91] Kondapalli LA, Perales-Puchalt A. Low birth weight: Is it related to assisted reproductive technology or underlying infertility? Fertility and Sterility. 2013; **99**(2):303-310

[92] McDonald SD et al. Preterm birth and low birth weight among in vitro fertilization twins: A systematic review and meta-analyses. European Journal of Obstetrics, Gynecology, and Reproductive Biology. 2010;**148**(2): 105-113

[93] McDonald SD et al. Preterm birth and low birth weight among in vitro fertilization singletons: A systematic review and meta-analyses. European Journal of Obstetrics, Gynecology, and Reproductive Biology. 2009;**146**(2): 138-148

[94] Statistics Canada. Health Fact Sheets Low Birth Weight Newborns in Canada. 2000–2013. Available from: https://www150.statcan.gc.ca/n1/pub/ 82-625-x/2016001/article/14674-eng. htm

[95] CDC. Percentage of Babies Born Low Birth Weight per State. 2018. Available from: https://www.cdc.gov/ nchs/pressroom/sosmap/lbw_births/ lbw.htm

[96] Wang YA et al. Preterm birth and low birth weight after assisted reproductive technology-related pregnancy in Australia between 1996 and 2000. Fertility and Sterility. 2005; **83**(6):1650-1658

[97] Schieve LA et al. Low and very low birth weight in infants conceived with use of assisted reproductive technology. The New England Journal of Medicine. 2002;**346**(10):731-737

[98] Sazonova A et al. Obstetric outcome after in vitro fertilization with single or double embryo transfer. Human Reproduction. 2011;**26**(2):442-450

[99] Henningsen AK et al. Perinatal outcome of singleton siblings born after assisted reproductive technology and spontaneous conception: Danish national sibling-cohort study. Fertility and Sterility. 2011;**95**(3):959-963

[100] Hayashi M et al. Adverse obstetric and perinatal outcomes of singleton pregnancies may be related to maternal factors associated with infertility rather than the type of assisted reproductive technology procedure used. Fertility and Sterility. 2012;**98**(4):922-928

[101] D'Angelo DV et al. Birth outcomes of intended pregnancies among women who used assisted reproductive technology, ovulation stimulation, or no treatment. Fertility and Sterility. 2011; **96**(2):314-320.e2

[102] Camarano L et al. Preterm delivery and low birth weight in singleton pregnancies conceived by women with and without a history of infertility. Fertility and Sterility. 2012;**98**(3): 681-686.e1

[103] Wisborg K, Ingerslev HJ, Henriksen TB. In vitro fertilization and preterm delivery, low birth weight, and admission to the neonatal intensive care unit: A prospective follow-up study.

Fertility and Sterility. 2010;**94**(6): 2102-2106

[104] Romundstad LB et al. Effects of technology or maternal factors on perinatal outcome after assisted fertilisation: A population-based cohort study. Lancet. 2008;**372**(9640):737-743

[105] Mitwally MF et al. Estradiol production during controlled ovarian hyperstimulation correlates with treatment outcome in women undergoing in vitro fertilization-embryo transfer. Fertility and Sterility. 2006; **86**(3):588-596

[106] Imudia AN et al. Peak serum estradiol level during controlled ovarian hyperstimulation is associated with increased risk of small for gestational age and preeclampsia in singleton pregnancies after in vitro fertilization. Fertility and Sterility. 2012;**97**(6): 1374-1379

[107] van der Spuy ZM et al. Outcome of pregnancy in underweight women after spontaneous and induced ovulation. British Medical Journal (Clinical Research Ed.). 1988;**296**(6627):962-965

[108] Cetin I, Cozzi V, Antonazzo P. Fetal development after assisted reproduction—A review. Placenta. 2003;**24**:S104-S113

[109] Kiserud T et al. The World Health Organization fetal growth charts: A multinational longitudinal study of ultrasound biometric measurements and estimated fetal weight. PLoS Medicine. 2017;**14**(1):e1002220

[110] Katalinic A et al. Pregnancy course and outcome after intracytoplasmic sperm injection: A controlled, prospective cohort study. Fertility and Sterility. 2004;**81**(6):1604-1616

[111] Jackson RA et al. Perinatal outcomes in singletons following

in vitro fertilization: A meta-analysis. Obstetrics and Gynecology. 2004; **103**(3):551-563

[112] Govement of the United Kingtom. Fertility Treatment in 2010: Trends and Figures by the Human Fertilisation and Embryology Authority. 2010 [cited 2018]. Available from: http://data.gov. uk/dataset/human-fertilisation-and-embryology-authority-fertility-treatment-2010-data

[113] Kramer MS. Born too small or too soon. The Lancet Global Health. 2013; **1**(1):e7-e8

[114] Gluckman PD et al. Effect of in utero and early-life conditions on adult health and disease. The New England Journal of Medicine. 2008;**359**(1):61-73

[115] Gluckman PD, Hanson MA. Developmental plasticity and human disease: Research directions. Journal of Internal Medicine. 2007;**261**(5):461-471

[116] Schieve LA et al. Does autism diagnosis age or symptom severity differ among children according to whether assisted reproductive technology was used to achieve pregnancy? Journal of Autism & Developmental Disorders. 2015;**45**(9): 2991-3003

[117] Wilson C, Pison G. More than half of the global population lives where fertility is below replacement level. Population and Societies. 2004;**405**:1-4

[118] Croen LA, Grether JK, Selvin S. Descriptive epidemiology of autism in a California population: Who is at risk? Journal of Autism and Developmental Disorders. 2002;**32**(3):217-224

[119] Haines L et al. UK population based study of severe retinopathy of prematurity: Screening, treatment, and outcome. Archives of Disease in

Childhood. Fetal and Neonatal Edition. 2005;**90**(3):F240-F244

[120] Keogh JM, Badawi N. The origins of cerebral palsy. Current Opinion in Neurology. 2006;**19**(2):129-134

[121] Surveillance of Cerebral Palsy in Europe (SCPE). Prevalence and characteristics of children with cerebral palsy in Europe. Developmental Medicine and Child Neurology. 2002; **44**(9):633-640

[122] Arneson CL et al. Prevalence of cerebral palsy: Autism and developmental disabilities monitoring network, three sites, United States, 2004. Disability and Health Journal. 2009;**2**(1):45-48

[123] Bhasin TK et al. Prevalence of four developmental disabilities among children aged 8 years—Metropolitan Atlanta Developmental Disabilities Surveillance Program, 1996 and 2000. MMWR Surveillance Summaries. 2006; **55**(1):1-9

[124] Paneth N, Hong T, Korzeniewski S. The descriptive epidemiology of cerebral palsy. Clinics in Perinatology. 2006;**33**(2):251-267

[125] Hvidtjorn D et al. Cerebral palsy, autism spectrum disorders, and developmental delay in children born after assisted conception: A systematic review and meta-analysis. Archives of Pediatrics & Adolescent Medicine. 2009;**163**(1):72-83

[126] Hvidtjorn D et al. Cerebral palsy among children born after in vitro fertilization: The role of preterm delivery—A population-based, cohort study. Pediatrics. 2006;**118**(2):475-482

[127] Klemetti R et al. Health of children born as a result of in vitro fertilization. Pediatrics. 2006;**118**(5):1819-1827

[128] Lidegaard O, Pinborg A, Andersen AN. Imprinting diseases and IVF:

Danish National IVF cohort study. Human Reproduction. 2005;**20**(4): 950-954

[129] Kallen B et al. In vitro fertilization in Sweden: Child morbidity including cancer risk. Fertility and Sterility. 2005; **84**(3):605-610

[130] Skrablin S et al. Long-term neurodevelopmental outcome of triplets. European Journal of Obstetrics, Gynecology, and Reproductive Biology. 2007;**132**(1):76-82

[131] Pinborg A et al. Morbidity in a Danish national cohort of 472 IVF/ICSI twins, 1132 non-IVF/ICSI twins and 634 IVF/ICSI singletons: Health-related and social implications for the children and their families. Human Reproduction. 2003;**18**(6):1234-1243

[132] Stromberg B et al. Neurological sequelae in children born after in-vitro fertilisation: A population-based study. Lancet. 2002;**359**(9305):461-465

[133] Pinborg A et al. Neurological sequelae in twins born after assisted conception: Controlled national cohort study. BMJ. 2004;**329**(7461):311

[134] Abdel-Latif ME et al. Neurodevelopmental outcomes of extremely premature infants conceived after assisted conception: A population based cohort study. Archives of Disease in Childhood. Fetal and Neonatal Edition. 2013;**98**(3):F205-F211

[135] Fountain C et al. Association between assisted reproductive technology conception and autism in California, 1997–2007. American Journal of Public Health. 2015;**105**(5): 963-971

[136] Sandin S et al. Autism and mental retardation among offspring born after in vitro fertilization. Journal of the American Medical Association. 2013; **310**(1):75-84

[137] Lehti V et al. Autism spectrum disorders in IVF children: A national case-control study in Finland. Human Reproduction. 2013;**28**(3):812-818

[138] Kamowski-Shakibai MT, Magaldi N, Kollia B. Parent-reported use of assisted reproduction technology, infertility, and incidence of autism spectrum disorders. Research in Autism Spectrum Disorders. 2015;**9**:77-95

[139] Mamidala MP et al. Maternal hormonal interventions as a risk factor for autism Spectrum disorder: An epidemiological assessment from India. Journal of Biosciences. 2013;**38**(5): 887-892

[140] Gillberg C, Wing L. Autism: Not an extremely rare disorder. Acta Psychiatrica Scandinavica. 1999;**99**(6): 399-406

[141] Christensen DL et al. Prevalence and characteristics of autism Spectrum disorder among children aged 8 years— Autism and developmental disabilities monitoring network, 11 sites, United States, 2012. MMWR Surveillance Summaries. 2016;**65**(3):1-23

[142] Boukhris T et al. Antidepressant use during pregnancy and the risk of autism spectrum disorder in children. JAMA Pediatrics. 2016;**170**(2):117-124

[143] Ackerman S et al. No increase in autism-associated genetic events in children conceived by assisted reproduction. Fertility & Sterility. 2014; **102**(2):388-393

[144] Lyall K et al. Fertility therapies, infertility and autism spectrum disorders in the Nurses' Health Study II. Paediatric and Perinatal Epidemiology. 2012;**26**(4):361-372

[145] Hediger ML et al. Assisted reproductive technologies and children's neurodevelopmental outcomes. Fertility and Sterility. 2013;**99**(2):311-317

[146] Association, A.P. Diagnostic and Statistical Manual of Mental Disorders. Fourth Edition: DSM-IV-TR®. American Psychiatric Association; 2000

[147] Association, A.P. Diagnostic and Statistical Manual of Mental Disorders. Fifth Edition: DSM-V. American Psychiatric Association; 2013

[148] Shojaei T et al. The strengths and difficulties questionnaire: Validation study in French school-aged children and cross-cultural comparisons. Social Psychiatry and Psychiatric Epidemiology. 2009;**44**(9):740-747

[149] McGrath JM et al. Parenting after infertility: Issues for families and infants. MCN: American Journal of Maternal Child Nursing. 2010;**35**(3): 156-164

[150] O'Connor TG et al. Maternal antenatal anxiety and behavioural/ emotional problems in children: A test of a programming hypothesis. Journal of Child Psychology and Psychiatry. 2003; **44**(7):1025-1036

[151] Talge NM, Neal C, Glover V. Antenatal maternal stress and long-term effects on child neurodevelopment: How and why? Journal of Child Psychology and Psychiatry. 2007;**48** (3–4):245-261

[152] O'Connor TG et al. Prenatal anxiety predicts individual differences in cortisol in pre-adolescent children. Biological Psychiatry. 2005;**58**(3): 211-217

[153] O'Connor TG, Heron J, Glover V. Antenatal anxiety predicts child behavioral/emotional problems independently of postnatal depression. Journal of the American Academy of Child and Adolescent Psychiatry. 2002; **41**(12):1470-1477

[154] Carson C et al. Effects of pregnancy planning, fertility, and assisted reproductive treatment on child

behavioral problems at 5 and 7 years: Evidence from the millennium cohort study. Fertility and Sterility. 2013;**99**(2): 456-463

[155] Golombok S et al. Families with children conceived by donor insemination: A follow-up at age twelve. Child Development. 2002;**73**(3):952-968

[156] Golombok S et al. Parent-child relationships and the psychological well-being of 18-year-old adolescents conceived by in vitro fertilisation. Human Fertility (Cambridge, England). 2009;**12**(2):63-72

[157] Wagenaar K et al. Behavior and socioemotional functioning in 9–18-year-old children born after in vitro fertilization. Fertility and Sterility. 2009;**92**(6):1907-1914

[158] Wagenaar K et al. Self-reported behavioral and socioemotional functioning of 11- to 18-year-old adolescents conceived by in vitro fertilization. Fertility and Sterility. 2011; **95**(2):611-616

[159] Zhu JL et al. Infertility, infertility treatment and behavioural problems in the offspring. Paediatric and Perinatal Epidemiology. 2011;**25**(5):466-477

[160] Brauner CB, Stephens CB. Estimating the prevalence of early childhood serious emotional/behavioral disorders: Challenges and recommendations. Public Health Reports. 2006;**121**(3):303-310

[161] Golombok S et al. Families created by the new reproductive technologies: Quality of parenting and social and emotional development of the children. Child Development. 1995;**66**(2):285-298

[162] Montgomery TR et al. The psychological status at school age of children conceived by in-vitro fertilization. Human Reproduction. 1999;**14**(8):2162-2165

Chapter 3

Oocyte Donation

Mehmet Musa Aslan

Abstract

Oocyte donations are ethical, social, religious, physiological, and medical problems. The medical risks of oocyte donation are not adequately addressed. The risks of oocyte donation require careful examination of the treatment of oocyte donors during the donation process. There are some long-term risks and various side effects such as pain, infection, oocyte retention, bleeding, premenstrual syndrome-like symptoms, ovarian hyperstimulation syndrome (OHSS), and the risk of ovarian cancer related to the drugs used by the donor. Treatment with oocyte donation is one of the situations in which the most common methods of assisted reproduction are discussed. There are many differences in moral, ethical, and religious issues in society. The use of donor eggs, sperm, or embryos is a social or cultural problem rather than a medical problem. For this reason, legal regulations on oocyte donation are carried out in line with cultural beliefs and public opinion about the procedure; individuals are free to use legal procedures according to their values. However, the fact that it is prohibited in some communities can push the illegal paths by obstructing the ones who want to use it.

Keywords: infertility, oocyte donation, fertility

1. Introduction

At the Universal Declaration of Human Rights, all women and men who reached adulthood—race, nationality, or religion without discrimination—have the right to establish a family. Reproductive and Sexual Rights Declaration also refers to "reproductive rights, sexual rights, and freedoms, as well as rights and freedoms that concern as much as individuals." The declaration drawn up by the International Declaration of Human Rights shows that sexual and reproductive rights are a legitimate part of basic human rights [1].

The family is of great importance in ensuring the continuation of the human race and in the training of the individuals suitable for the expectations of the society. Reproductive function is a universal function peculiar to individuals and families. Especially in traditional societies, the role of women in the family and society has been handled in connection with fertility and child care. The female reproductive organs, together with birth, give the individual a role of feminine and the girl child is prepared with this role in the future. As long as the reproductive organs are healthy, they give meaning to the life of the woman; social and psychological balance [2].

Establishing a family, being a child is a desirable condition accepted in all societies. The development of the society and the continuation of the generations depend on it [3]. Having family and children is the primary and social duty of the individual. The infertile woman, while accepting it, violates the norms of behavior by not being a child. Just like in all world societies, in Turkish society, marriage brings together the possession of children and problems arise in marriages where the child is not. After the marriage, the childless family is unthinkable and the couple is expected to have children immediately [4].

For infertile couples who cannot have children as they wish, the situation is very difficult; because infertility is a process that is tiring, weary, time, labor, and money for diagnosis and treatment. Moreover, infertility may cause women to consider themselves less valuable and insufficient [5].

Infertility, which causes biological, psychological, psychosocial, and culturally important problems in infertile couples, is the inability of the couples in the reproductive age to become pregnant or to continue the gestation [6–9], even though they have sexual intercourse three to four times a week for 1 year.

Having children in Islamic societies is an important goal for marriage and seems to be very important for the stability and happiness of marriage life. For this reason, infertile couples who cannot achieve this basic tendency tend to be judged by the society as unsuccessful. In this context, infertility is an important social problem that can affect relationships and even threaten marriage. In addition, the social environment makes the situation even more difficult by bringing couples into contact with community expectations [10].

Today, there are a variety of treatment options for infertility, and new technologies are emerging to address this important health problem affecting about 15–20% of married couples. There are a number of assisted reproduction models, some of which are carried out by third parties such as gametes or embryo donations and carrier maternity. Women with ovarian failure were considered irreversibly sterile until about 20 years ago, but this view has changed as they have developed in assisted reproductive techniques (ART). Today, women with premature ovarian failure or fast ovarian reserve can be given a realistic pregnancy chance by oocyte donation. Oocyte donation is often carried out by In vitro fertilization (IVF) after ovarian hyperstimulation is controlled, followed by transfer of sperm to the uterus of recipient from the oocyte transporter partner, a healthy young donor. Using donated oocytes, the first successful pregnancy in a recipient woman was performed in 1983 [11]. It is now a developing area of oocyte donation assisted reproductive technology.

Treatment with oocyte donation is one of the most controversial aspects of assisted reproduction. There are many differences of opinion in moral, ethical, and religious matters in society. It can be estimated that oocyte donation is even more complicated in Islamic societies when it is thought that by the third parties even the proselytizing is considered unacceptable in some Islamic rules according to some people and that the legislation prohibits it. Many countries have begun to donate oocytes by making the necessary legal arrangements in line with their values and beliefs. The rights of donor, recipient couple, and child are guaranteed by these laws. Frequently adopted adoptions before ART appear to be a solution to the problem of infertile people, but they are inadequate when considering blood and racial prevalence and can cause psychological problems in parents and children. In Anatolia, an attempt has been made to find a solution in the form of adoption of nephews in the family by taking into consideration the adoption of blood and racial preoccupation. Adoption is the biological link that the ART can provide and the lack of enthusiasm for having a child remains an undesirable option. In Islam, some schools prohibit the adoption of other than the father's [12].

One of the problems brought by assisted reproductive therapy is who is the real parent of the child. Unless third-party genetic material is used, there is no confusion in the concepts of mother and father. For this reason, the use of genetic material by third parties in the implementation of ART in religious traditions and in the laws of most countries is not tolerated [13].

Donor egg, sperm, or embryo use is a social or cultural problem rather than a medical problem. For this reason, legal regulations on oocyte donations, cultural beliefs, and community are made in line with procedural considerations; individuals are free to use legal procedures according to their own values. However, the fact that it is prohibited in some communities can push them to illegal ways by preventing those who want to use it. Infertile couples try to find solutions for both infertility and other adverse effects, and try a variety of treatment options.

2. General information

2.1 Infertility

2.1.1 History

Reproduction is a concept that has been very important since ancient times. Initially, thinkers who lived in ancient times carried out their efforts to understand the human reproductive system and the dysfunctions in this system, after which the scientists continued their work on this subject. The first texts about infertility date back to 2200–1950 BC. Hippocrates, who lived between 460 and 370 BC, also mentioned infertility [14]. The prescriptions for the early recognition of pregnancy and the prevention of infertility were first used in ancient Egypt [15].

The first artificial fertilization in the world was obtained by Hunter between 1776 and 1799 [14–16]. The first reference to reproductive dates back to antiquity, and one of the first examples is the biblical command, "be productive and multiplicative." According to religious beliefs, God was the source of both fertility and infertility. A woman's ability to raise children is considered as a measure of her femininity; infertility was seen as a punishment of misconduct [14–16].

Rapid developments in reproductive health in the past 30 years have also increased interest and expectation for the concept of infertility. The definition of infertility was accepted in recent years although the couple in reproductive age has been unprotected, sexually related three to four times a week for at least a year [17–20]. It is suggested that infertility rate in the world affects more than 80 million people in the world, which is seen in different ratios in different countries, and it is stated that the infertility rate varies between 5 and 30%.

In industrialized societies, it is estimated that 10–15% of couples receive a primary or secondary infertility diagnosis. This ratio increases to 30–50% in African countries [21]. Turkey is also considered a diagnosis of infertility in 10–20% of couples [20, 21]. Increased infertility due to various factors all over the world is seen as a developmental crisis involving individual and spousal relationships rather than a medical situation due to the emotional problems created in individuals and marriage relations.

2.1.2 Reproduction process and infertility

In order for the breeding period to be successfully completed, the male and female physiology must have the maturation and conditions necessary for reproduction. Firstly, hypothalamus-Pituitary aksis, fallopian tube functions, cervical and endometrial conditions; and hypothalamic-hypophyseal-testicular axis in men, sperm production, and mobility should be normal [22, 23].

2.1.3 Incidence of infertility

Infertility is a question of varying frequency and cause of region to region, involving 15% of men and women in the reproductive age [24]. According to the survey, South Korea (1.3%), Jordan (2.2%), and Syria (2.9%) were the lowest in the 40–49 age group. In contrast, especially in Africa, some tribes and communities have much higher rates of infertility. For example, 65% of women aged 45–49 in Mbelo in Zaire are without children [25]. Health care practitioners in the United States report that the incidence of infertility is 15%, that is, it affects one in every six pairs or 4.8 million women [26].

According to the results of the 1990 census in our country, the rate of married women aged 15–49 is 23%, which is calculated as 11.3 million women. When the incidence of infertility is accepted as 8.5%, it corresponds to 1.5 million women and consequently it directly affects at least 3 million people. This is a large population that is longing for children. According to the results of the 1993 census, the proportion of women who say that it is not possible to give birth at all is found to be 9.5% [26].

3. Infertility reasons and treatment

Clinically, there are two forms of infertility, physiological and pathological infertility. Infertile pairs; 40–55% infertility is the cause of women, 25–40% in men, 10% in both, and 10% in cases of unexplained reason.

Causes of infertility due to females are: 30–40% ovulatory dysfunction, 30–40% tubal peritoneal factor, 10–15% unexplained infertility, and 10–15% multiple factors together [12, 27]. While 15% of married couples have infertility, only 1–2% have sterility. There is a certain height of reasons for the woman here, because after the ejaculation, the function of the man ends for fertilization. Fertility, however, is not finished here but has just begun [26].

3.1 Causes of physiological infertility

Causes of physiological infertility are: infantile infertility, pregnancy infertility, lactation infertility, postmenopausal infertility, cyclic infertility, voluter infertility, and relative and social infertility.

a. **Infantile infertility**: infertility is seen in this period because it is not usually a reproductive function at 12–15 years old.

b. **Pregnancy infertility**: a pregnant woman cannot conceive a second time during her pregnancy.

c. **Lactation infertility**: some women may not conceive as long as they are breastfeeding.

d. **Postmenopausal infertility**: reproduction stops with the end of ovarian functions.

e. **Cyclic infertility**: 28–30 days of normal cycle, ovulation occurs on the 14th or 15th day. After 8 h of ovulation, the chances of fecundity will decrease every hour and will rise within 24 h. Except for days 10–17 of the cycle, the woman is physiologically infertile

f. **Voluter infertility**: infertility is the result of the wishes of couples not having children with their own desire.

g. **Relative and social infertility**: marriage is not regular and healthy when married couples are ill after marriage, military service, college, work situation, etc. The infertility that occurs in these conditions is called relative and social infertility [7, 28, 29]. All infertile pathologies other than physiological infertility are pathologically infertile. It is possible to collect the causes of pathological infertility under three large groups.

3.2 Causes of pathological infertility

Causes of pathological infertility are general causes, extragenital causes, and genital causes.

3.2.1 Common causes

Infertility affects intellectual, sexual mismatch, obesity, drug dependence, hypovitaminosis, protein deficiency, iron deficiency anemia, stress, excessive alcohol, coffee and cigarette intake, radiation, and heavy metal poisoning [7, 12].

3.2.2 Extragenital causes

1. **Hypophyseal**: increase or decrease of pituitary function causes secondary failure. Hypopituitarism, hemorrhagic circulation collapse and pituitary necrosis (Sheehan syndrome), granulomas, cysts, tumors, galactorrhea, amenorrhea syndromes, hunger, and anemia may result [7, 12, 29].

2. **Thyroid**: hypothyroidism—anovulation, infertility, and abortion; and hyperthyroidism—amenorrhea causes infertility if severe.

3. **Adrenal**: adrenocortical hyperfunction (Cushing's disease) weakens ovulation and adrenal insufficiency (Addison's disease) causes gonadal atrophy.

3.2.3 Genital causes

Genital causes of the female according to the organs [7, 26, 29]:

1. Causes of vulva and vagina

2. Causes of cervical

3. Causes of uterus

4. Causes of tuba uterine

5. Over hypothalamus and hypophthalmia causes

6. Metabolic diseases and other causes

7. Psychic causes

3.2.4 Genital causes of men

Factors that cause infertility in men are less than in women. Male infertility factors are abnormal spermatogenesis, abnormal motility, anatomical disorders, endocrine disorders, and sexual dysfunction. Anatomical abnormalities are probably caused by congenital absence of vas deferens, vas deferens obstruction, and abnormalities of the ejaculatory system. Abnormal spermatogenesis may develop due to mumps orchid, chromosomal abnormalities, cryptorchidism, chemical or radiation exposure, and varicocele [12]. Excessive temperature exposure, severe allergic reaction, exposure to radiation and environmental toxins, high amounts of narcotic drugs, and alcohol and drug use significantly affect sperm quality and number [30]. Immunity can play a role in some infertility. Antisperm antibodies were found in 72% of infertile couples in males and in 13% of females. It has been suggested that all antibodies against sperm may play a role in infertility by inhibiting sperm cervical mucus penetration by reducing sperm motility in the female genital tract by causing agglutination, immobilization, or opsonization [26, 31].

3.3 Evaluation of infertile couples

Infertile couples should be examined and treated together. Infertile couples are examined by anamnesis, general examination, and laboratory studies, and five cardinal examinations are performed after genital examinations. These examinations are performed on certain days of the menstrual cycle, and none of them have priority over the others [24, 29, 32, 33].

1. Spermiogram

2. Ovulation detection

3. Hysterosalpingography

4. Postcoital test

5. Laparoscopy

3.3.1 Anamnesis

Couples should be evaluated together and a good history should be taken. The history is very important. With a good history, about 50% is diagnosed. Sometimes 100% is diagnosed and verified by examinations.
Information necessary to take in the history:

- Age and duration of marriage (the prognosis is poor since the ovarian reserve is over 35 years old) and duration of infertility

- Previous pregnancy, low number of cases, any complication of pregnancy, and menstrual history (such as menarche age, duration of menstruation, frequency, and order)

- Previous infertility tests and treatments

- Whether there are diseases such as lung, heart, kidney disease, or urogenital disease

- Sexual history (frequency, timing, vaginismus, dyspareunia)

- Occupational and environmental life, chemical or radiation containing substances, hobbies, and work habits [4, 24, 34]

3.3.2 General examination

Female genitourinary and pelvic examination is assessed for congenital anomaly, abnormal uterine position, pelvic pathology (such as endometriosis, ovarian cysts, and myomas), and vaginal discharge. It should be emphasized whether it is sexual or hirsutismus. In addition, the development status of the breasts and the presence of galactorrhea should be investigated [26, 35]. An infertile man should also be examined by a specialist andrologist and urologist. The condition of testes and the examination of the epididymis and ductus deferens should be performed to check whether varicocele is present [29, 35, 36].

3.3.3 Special examinations

This includes semen analysis in men, ultrasonography, endocrine tests, testicular biopsy, and sperm penetration tests. Postovulatory tests, ultrasonography, endometrial biopsy, hysterosalpingography, hysteroscopy, laparoscopy, and endocrine tests are included determining the day of ovulation.

Tests for man:

- Spermiogram

- Endocrine tests

- Ultrasonography

- Testicular biopsy

- Sperm penetration test

Tests for women:

- Ovulation detection

- Basal body temperature

- Serum progesterone measurements

- Endometrial biopsy

- Examination of cervical mucus

- Ultrasonography

- Hysterosalpingography

- Laparoscopy

3.4 Surgical treatment of infertility

Treatment of varicocele in men is to remove obstruction by minimally invasive method in male or female, myomectomy, hysteroscopy or metroplasty in some anomalies, intrauterine synechia, septum or polyps hysteroscopy. In addition, in cases of endometriosis not resolved with medical treatment and retrogradation in extreme cases, laparotomy or laparoscopy is performed [1, 4, 26]. Tubal or pelvic causes caused by pelvic inflammatory disease (PID) can be corrected by microsurgical techniques or by performing laparotomy for the opening of pelvic adhesions [35]. To correct the coital factor, psychotherapy, sexual therapy, and artificial insemination are applied with sperm of partner [1].

4. Assisted reproduction techniques

Assisted reproductive techniques are a general concept and include many methods. Assisted reproductive techniques (ART) are the names given to procedures performed following ovarian oocyte retrieval [9, 37, 38].

4.1 Intrauterine insemination (artificial insemination, IUI)

The insertion of spermatozoa into the genital tract without coitus is called insemination. If the cervix is placed, that is, if cervical insemination is placed into the uterus cavity, it is called intrauterine insemination; and if placed in a peritoneal cavity, it is called peritoneal insemination. Insemination with sperm taken from a woman's wife is called homologous insemination, whereas insemination with sperm taken from another man is called insemination. There is no donor insemination (DI) in our country according to the law. The success rate for intrauterine insemination (IUI) is 10–15% [24, 39].

4.2 In vitro fertilization and embryo transfer (IVF-ET)

The oocyte matured with a needle guided by laparoscopy or transcervical ultrasonography is aspirated from the ovary. Spermatozoids from the man are placed in tissue culture in the laboratory. After fertilization has occurred, the ovum is placed in the uterus of the embryo at the morula stage (4–16 cell stage) [1, 12, 24, 36, 40]. The optimal period for transfer is 48–72 h after insemination [2].

4.3 Gamete intrafallopian transfer (GIFT)

The basic principle in the gamete intrafallopian transfer method is that eggs were developed by controlled hyperthermia and aspirated and put into the tuba ampulla with the sperm. In order to apply GIFT, it is necessary and sufficient that at least one tubane detected by permeability hysterosalpingography is open. The success rate in GIFT is 20–30% [3, 24, 39, 41]. Gamete intrafallopian transfer has the advantage over the IVF method; the reason for the application of the method under laparoscopy is that the 2-day laboratorial incubation period and the embryo's placement into the uterine cavity have been eliminated. The disadvantage of the method is the individual must have to work fast during anesthesia and the application of the laboratory's method [26, 39].

4.4 Intracytoplasmic sperm injection (microinjection, ICSI)

It is placed in the oocyte cytoplasm with a sperm micropipette. ICSI can be used not only in cases with very low sperm counts but also in gamete interferences in zona pellucida and vitelline membrane level. ICSI has also been used successfully in qualitative, functional sperm disorders and idiopathic infertility cases [24, 26, 42].

4.5 Zygote intrafallopian transfer (ZIFT)

Oocyte and sperm are fertilized in vitro, and then zygote is injected into the tuba bulb by laparoscopy [24]. But this is not implemented today.

5. Assisted reproduction techniques and ethics

Thanks to advances in medical technology, people have had the opportunity to change this evil fate. As well as having evil in every good, the ART has brought religious, legal, and ethical problems together. The main opposition line against the ART is representative of religious traditions. The belief and acceptance system, which takes an important place in the formation of social consensus, derives from religious traditions [43].

Concentration of theologians and religious thinkers on the ethical and scientific aspects of assisted reproductive technology can be evaluated in four overlapping periods. The first period covers the mid-1960s. The initial debate is the defense of genetics and biologists who consider clearing the gene pool from defective genes through selected genotypes based on reproductive control, alternative ART, and cloning [44, 45]. Protestant Josef Fletcher, who participated in the debate in this period, defended the increase of control over human autonomy and human repro-duction. Paul Ramsey, a Protestant, also treats the ART as a "border" and regards it as a situation that must be chosen between humanity and creation at risk. Ramsey predicted three horizontal (human-human) and two vertical (human-god) bound-aries in the ART and defined them as the point of passage.

1. ART reproduction: (or tried to be) gene pool.

2. Second ART: it will include nontherapeutic research on unborn babies.

3. Third ART: it will transform "creation" into "reproductive" which will affect the parental concept, which will harm the unifying and creative aspects of the sexual outcome [44, 46].

Vertical boundaries are:

1. **Assisted reproduction**: he is carrying the sin of eternal vanity.

2. **Assisted reproduction**: The second period began in 1978 with two important events. The first in vitro fertilization product was published by Louise Brown and David Rorvik's book [44, 45]. The basis of ethical advocacy of assisted reproduction technology is the use of the reproductive right of the person. If a

person uses this right for contraception, he can also use it for the right to have children. The right to reproduction includes not only the "child" ownership of the person but also the physical and mental health of the child. If there is genetic disease that can be transmitted through the body, efforts to prevent this transmission are ethically and legally acceptable [29]. Adoptive adoption before the development of assisted reproduction technology appears to be a solution to the problem of infertile people, but it is inadequate especially in Muslim and Jewish societies when blood and nesseben prevalence is considered and can cause psychological problems in parents and children. In Anatolia, an attempt was made to find a solution in the form of adoption of nests in the family by taking the blood-bondage and the nesseben advantage of adoption. Adoption is the biological link that the ART can provide, and the lack of enthusiasm for having a child remains an undesirable option. In Islam, some schools ban men from adopting children, so that one can be regarded as someone other than his father [12].

One of the problems brought by assisted reproductive technology is who is the real parent of the child. Unless the third-party genetic material is used, there is no confusion in the concepts of mother and father. For this reason, the use of genetic material by third parties in the implementation of the ART in religious traditions and in the laws of most countries is not tolerated [46]. Religious traditions have emphasized the family institution and the sanctity of love. The unity of love and the creative nature manifest itself in the birth of a baby. The care and growth of this child belongs to the blessed family institution. Any event that will shake the structure of the family will affect the development of the child's personality. Because ART will affect family morals and religious roles, the basic structure of the family will also be affected. The ART regulation in force in our country has only allowed married couples to serve this issue [47].

Some countries and regions have legally accepted sperm and oocyte donations. Artificial insemination donor "AID" is called artificial insemination applied with sperm supplied from sperm banks. In this case, the name of the donor is kept secret. With this technique, who will be the father of the child born after pregnancy? How much love can this child be able to adopt to his wife? If the spouses cannot agree and divorce, can the father-in-law reject the spouse? [8].

When assisted reproductive technology is applied, it may be the mechanization of sexual intercourse. The couple may look at treatment as a method against performance inadequacy, rather than just medical intervention, which can lead to feelings of guilt, unconscious indictments, and serious ego trauma in the responsible person [4]. With the material from the third person, with the help of the ART, it is possible to marry two brothers who are unaware of each other, which creates great danger for the generations. Maternity is one of the main causes in a woman's life. Today, the definition of traditional motherhood, "giving birth to blood and bringing up children" has become debatable, and "bonding with love," genetic motherhood has the same prescription [6]. For many, life begins with the fertilization of the egg; no matter how early the embryo is a human offspring. Putting him in a fridge like an inanimate object, doing experiments on it, and eventually throwing it in a waste basket is neither moral nor faithful [41, 48].

Oxford scientist Prof. Dr. Warnaek reflected his worries: societies have some rules and boundaries about their lives and their treatment of their deaths, loyalty and respect, honor, and sexual life. These limits and rules may vary from community to community, as well as from time to time in the same community. However, if a society totally loses its own principles, this is the problem of morality for that society. For this reason, lawmakers, philosophers, and scholars limit new developments

[49]. Along with the development of in vitro fertilization techniques, problems such as the establishment of sperm banks, the beginning of sperm business, the surplus of frozen embryos, and rental motherhood have been accompanied. Companies selling egg cells, sperm-cell-trading companies, bring about results like desperately attempting to influence the gender of the fetus, big irregularities, children born disabled, or sexually ill. The most controversial issue arising from in vitro fertilization is the situation of fertilized egg. Collection of eggs occurs with oocyte pick-up (OPU) process. The chance of successful fertilization and cellular division is increasing statistically by taking more than one ovum and making more than one fertilization. With medical induction technique, more eggs are formed and several eggs are taken and fertilized. During the resetting procedure in practice, more than one fertilized egg is transferred to the offspring of the mother and this raises the risk of multiple pregnancies. Some problems arise during this process. Although the first problem requires a moral ground, this is the legal direction. The European Union is taking the protection of embryos in vitro through the 1997 Oviedo Convention on Human Rights. Accordingly, it is forbidden to produce human embryos for research purposes [52].

Contrary to organ donors, gamete donors are likely to survive when used for egg or sperm fertilization. It is not lawful to accept the right to use gamete cells as an acquired right as it is in fertilized human eggs. The donation of gametes used in fertilization from moral, religious, and social care should not be considered as an ordinary cell donation [53]. Religious views and beliefs constitute the moral foundations of society. The religious beliefs and beliefs of the community play an important role in the formation of social norms in almost all societies around the world. Social norms draw a basic philosophical framework of how life should be experienced. The fundamental resistance to the ART comes from religious men and thinkers. The reason is that assisted reproductive technology destroys ongoing social norms and assumptions [3, 9]. The tube was the ideal research material for embryo scientists in the refrigerator. Many dark spots of science have given birth to daylight. Thus, it is possible to examine the metabolism of the human embryo and to know which substances are useful and which substances are harmful [55]. Another fact that limits the ART is that individual benefit is the priority rather than social benefit. Preliminary screening of individual benefit is an effort to prevent genetic discrimination [46, 50, 51].

It is not possible to solve and clarify any complicated problems with animal experiments. Thalidomide, which is harmless in animals, was used in humans in the 1960s and caused the birth of thousands of people without sleeves [51]. Although the embryo is not legally regarded as a full personality, it must be treated with reverence. An inanimate object should be treated like a human fetus, not as a piece of furniture. Otherwise, this may slowly lead people to newborns, comatose patients, change their attitudes toward the elderly, and lose their respect. The embryo is mistaken to look like a complete human being. Moreover, it should not be forgotten that researches on embryos will make a great contribution to humanity. In this sense, it is not possible to give up. As technologists progress, customs do not always stay in the same place. Their change is also awaited [43]. This slogan "to play God" is most often and often expressed in the critique of medical developments. The concerns expressed with this slogan are very diverse. It is thought that people should not investigate the mysteries of life. The scientific explanations of these mysteries are: it can lead to the creation of a theology of thought that includes mysteries unexplainable in humans only by the concept of "God filling in the gaps" which is explained by the dogmas of religion [54].

Diseases related to sex can be prevented by performing gender determination in embryos, and the formation of mongol babies can be prevented by performing chromosome examination. Improvement of metabolism has been detected at the growth phase of the embryo by reduction of the material called pyruvate. With the same experience, the penetrating ability of the sperm was multiplied and it is now possible to fertilize oligospermia cases with less than 2 million sperms in cm^3 [46]. The embryos used in all these experiments also go to the waste basket. This is causing great objections. For many, life begins with the fertilization of your egg; no matter how early the embryo is human, the fetus [55]. IVF can lead to some dangerous developments, and these developments can be economic, esthetic, and political; for example, attempts to create superior races [51].

The evaluation of the effects of new techniques on subsequent generations is very important. This is investigated by studies on other species and investigated as limited use in clinical trials. Chromosomal assays in the 8-cell and blastocyst stage of the human embryo provide a new technique for evaluating the adverse effects of new techniques. The defense of the artificial nature of this new technique emphasizes that all medical treatments are artificial and aim at correcting the mistakes of nature [51].

Author details

Mehmet Musa Aslan
Department of Obstetrics and Gynecology, Sakarya University Education and Research Hospital, Sakarya, Turkey

*Address all correspondence to: jinopdrmma@gmail.com

IntechOpen

References

[1] Asena A. NMS Gynecology and Obstetrics. İstanbul: Nobel Bookstore; 1998. pp. 359-364

[2] Çolgar V. In vitro fertilization and embryo transfer. Journal of Gynecology and Obstetrics. 1998:73-81

[3] Akyüz A. Nursing in adaptation to IVF treatment [Doctoral thesis]. Ankara, T.C.: General Staff Gülhane Military Medical Academy Institute of Health Sciences; 2001

[4] AK G. Depression situations of infertile couples and investigation of their initiation paths [Master thesis]. İzmir: Dokuz Eylül University, Institute of Health Sciences; 2001

[5] Temizel N. Determination of the Status of Women Attending IVF-ET Center. II. National Nursing Congress Reports. İzmir: Ege University, Medical Faculty Hospital; 1990. pp. 801-808

[6] Scherrod RA. Coping with infertility a personal perspective turned professional. MCN: American Journal of Maternal Child Nursing. 1988;13(3):191-194

[7] Şirin A. A study on socio-demographic characteristics and nurses' expectations of hospitalized patients for IVF-ET. Health Services Vocational School Journal İstanbul University. 1998;4(4):27-34

[8] Valentin DP. Psychological impact of infertility identifying issues and needs. Social Work in Health Care. 1986;11(4):61-69

[9] Vural B. Yücesoy İ, Erk A. Karabacak O. Assisted reproductive techniques. 1999;46-53.

[10] Kırca N, Pasinlioğlu T. Psychosocial problems encountered in infertility treatment. Current Approaches in Psychiatry. 2013;5(2):162-178

[11] Tsai MC, Takeuchi T, Bedford JM, Reis MM, Rosenwaks Z, Palermo GD. Opinion: Alternative sources of gametes: Reality or science fiction? Human Reproduction. 2000;15(5):98898

[12] Işık AZ, Vicdan K. Clinical Gynecology and Endocrinology Handbook; 2003. pp. 431-469

[13] Rainsbury PA, Viniker DA. In: Işık AZ, Vicdan K, Atabeyoğlu L, editors. Practical Approaches to Reproductive Medicine. Ankara: Atlas Bookstore; 1998. pp. 279-293

[14] Morice P, Josset P, Dubuisson JB. History of sterility in ancient times. I. Sterility in Egypt. Diagnostic recipes for sterility and pregnancy in ancient Egypt. Contraception, Fertilité, Sexualité (1992). 1995;23:423-427

[15] Bateman-Cass CS. The Loss within A Loss: Understanding the Psychological Implications of Assisted Reproductive Technologies for the Treatment of Infertility. San Diego: California School of Professional Psychology; 2000

[16] Erdem Atak İR. Unexplained infertility is the transmission of maternal mothers and females [thesis]. İstanbul: İstanbul University, Social Sciences Institute; 2009

[17] Lohrmann JA. A psychological investigation of women's experience of successfully coping with infertility [Unpublished Doctor of Philosophy thesis]. 1995

[18] Yanıkkerem E, Kavlak O, Sevil Ü. Problems of infertile couples and nursing approach. Ataturk University School of Nursing Journal. 2008;11:112-121

[19] Taşçı E, Bolsoy N, Kavlak O, Yücesoy F. Marriage adaptation in

infertile women. Turkish Society of Gynecology and Obstetrics. 2008;5:105-110

[20] Eren N. The impact of perceived social support on infertility-related stress and marital adjustment in infertile couples [thesis]. Ankara: Gazi University, Faculty of Medicine, Department of Psychiatry; 2008

[21] Ramazanzadeh F, Noorbala AA, Abedinia N, Naghizadeh MM. Emotional adjustment in infertile couples: Systematic review article. Iranian Journal of Reproductive Medicine. 2009;7:97-103

[22] Akerer B. 15-49 Yaş Kadınların Jinekolojik Muayene Öncesi Anksiyete Durumlarının İncelenmesi [Tez]. İzmir: Ege Üniversitesi, Sağlık Bilimleri Enstitüsü; 2003

[23] Reeder SJ, Martin LL, Koıak-Griftin D. Maternity Nursing Family, Newborn. 18th ed. Lippincott Company; 1997. pp. 319-338

[24] Yıldırım M. Clinical Infertility. 2nd ed. Ankara: Eryılmaz Printing Press; 2000. pp. 31-39; 299-306

[25] Akyüz A, İnanç N. Nursing in in vitro fertilization. Syndrome. 1998:128-131

[26] Kavlak O. The loneliness level in infertile women and the factors affecting it [Doctoral thesis]. İzmir: Ege University, Health Sciences Institute, Nursing High School; 1999

[27] Family Planning Clinical Practice Manual Book. İstanbul: T.C. Ministry of Health, General Directorate of Mother and Child Health and Family Planning, Human Resource Development Foundation; 1997. pp. 251-262

[28] Terzioğlu F, Sandak F, Kılıç S. Determination of anxiety levels of cows participating in assisted reproductive

technology. In: II. National Clinician Nurses and Ebeler Congress; Antalya; 2001

[29] Şirin A. Lectures on Women's Diseases and Nursing. İzmir; 2002. pp. 355-364

[30] İbrahimoğlu L, Yüksel A, Alkış R, Ermiş H, Deniz Y. Place of genital tuberculosis in cases of infertility. Journal of Obstetrics and Gynecology. 1989;3:38-41

[31] Seyisoğlu H, Erel TC, İrez T, Eren T, Ertüngealp E. Clinical value of antisperm antibody in infertile women. Journal of Obstetrics and Gynecology. 1995;9:41-45

[32] Yıldırım M. Clinical Gynecology. Ankara: Contemporary Medical Publishing; 1992. pp. 68-89

[33] Ünal MT, Sağlam K, Kutlu M. Evaluation of infertile couples. JAMA. 1992:24-29

[34] Gürgan T, Demirol A. Overview of infertility. Actual Medical Journal Special Issue on Women's Health. 2001;6(1):52-55

[35] Dervişoğlu AA. Contraceptive Methods. Ankara: International Printing; 1990. pp. 139-165

[36] Şirin A. The Practice of In Vitro Fertilization and the Approach to Couples from this Application. İzmir; 2001

[37] Jirka J, Schuettfoxall MJ. Lonelinnes and social support in infertile couples. Journal of Obstetric, Gynecologic, and Neonatal Nursing. 1996;25(1):55-59

[38] Jhonson CL. Self esteem: Strategies and invention for the infertile women. Journal of Obstetric, Gynecologic, and Neonatal Nursing. 1996;25(4):291-295

[39] Terzioğlu F. Determination of counseling needs of nursing mothers

and examination of the efficiency of nurses' counseling service [thesis]. Ankara: Hacettepe University, Institute of Health Sciences; 1998

[40] Günalp S, Erçakmak S. Diagnosis of Obstetrics and Gynecology. Ankara; 1998. pp. 210-215

[41] İdil M. Assisted reproductive methods and gift. Obstetrics Gynecology Continuing Education Journal. 1997;**1**(3,4):303-310

[42] Turan C, Gökmen O, Doğan M, Keleş G, Uygun M, Çelikkanat H, et al. Pregnancy loss rates in ICSI and IVF pregnancies. Obstetrics and Gynecology New Views and Developments. 1998;**10**(1):62-64

[43] Dhillan R, Cumming CE, Cumming DC. Psychological well-being and coping patterns in infertile men. Fertility and Sterlity. 2000;**747**(2):702-706

[44] Hirch MA, Hirch MS. The long-term psychosocial effects of infertility. Journal of Obstetric, Gynecologic, and Neonatal Nursing. 1995;**24**(6):517-522

[45] Family Planning Clinical Practice Handbook. İstanbul: T. C. Ministry of Health, General Directorate of Mother and Child Health and Family Planning, Human Resources Development Foundation; 1997. pp. 251-262

[46] Rainsbury PA, Viniker DA. In: Işık AZ, Vicdan K, Atabeyoğlu L, editors. Üreme Tıbbına Pratik Yaklaşımlar [Çeviren]. Ankara: Atlas Kitapçılık; 1998. pp. 279-293

[47] Dalaner H. Examination of state-continuity anxiety levels before and after inseminating feminine insemination [thesis]. Izmir: Ege University, Health Sciences Institute; 2000

[48] Urman B. Case selection and application indications in assisted reproductive technology. Obstetrics and Gynecology Continuing Education Journal. 1997;**1**:311-323

[49] Family Planning Clinical Practice Handbook. T. C. Ministry of Health, General Directorate of Mother and Child Health and Family Planning, President Ayşe Akın Dervişoğlu, Nobel Medical Books; 1995

[50] Türkoğlu D, Tamam L, Evlice YE. Psychiatric aspects of infertility. Thinking Man. 1997;**10**(4):48-54

[51] Regulation of nursing assisted treatment centers. Ministry of Health General Directorate of Mother and Child Health and Family Planning; 2005

[52] Guz H, Ozkan A, Sarisoy G, Yanik F, Yanik A. Psychiatric symptoms in Turkish infertile women. Journal of Psychosomatic Obstetrics and Gynecology. 2003;**24**:267-271

[53] Milliard S. Emotional response to infertility understanding patients need's. AORN Journal. 1991;**54**(2):301-305

[54] Davis DC, Dearman CN. Coping strategies of infertile women. Journal of Obstetric, Gynecologic, and Neonatal Nursing. 1991;**20**(3):221-228

[55] Doğan M, Terazi A. Infertility nursing entrance and infertility policlinic services. THD. 1990;**39**:4

Chapter 4

Cryopreservation of Oocytes and Embryos: Current Status and Opportunities

Arindam Dhali, Atul P. Kolte, Ashish Mishra, Sudhir C. Roy and Raghavendra Bhatta

Abstract

The biochemical and metabolic activities of living cells are virtually stopped at ultralow temperature and they enter into a suspended state of animation. However, as such, exposure of living cells to ultralow temperature is associated with complex changes that reduce their survivability following freeze-thawing. Cryopreservation is the method for preserving living cells at ultralow temperature at genetically and physiologically stabilized state. Cryopreservation of oocytes and embryos is an integral part of the assisted reproductive technologies with many potential applications. Cryobanking of oocytes and embryos derived from genetically superior animals is promising for enhancing the outcome of planned breeding programs and conserving biodiversity of endangered animal species. Cryobanking can also ensure steady supply of oocytes and embryos for many downstream applications of assisted reproduction such as in vitro embryo production, embryo transfer, production of stem cells, and genetic engineering. Tremendous advancements have been made in this field over the past 5 decades and several methods have been demonstrated for cryopreserving oocytes and embryos in different species. This chapter focuses on the fundamental aspects of oocyte and embryo cryopreservation.

Keywords: cryopreservation, oocyte, embryo, methods, challenges

1. Introduction

The extent of metabolic processes and cellular functions of living cells are reduced dramatically in response to low temperature [1]. Further, at ultralow temperature, the biochemical and metabolic activities of living cells are virtually stopped and they enter into a suspended state of animation. Nevertheless, the exposure of living cells to ultralow temperature induces complex changes to the cells that are associated with its altered physical structure and biophysical processes. These facts indicate that living cells can be preserved at ultralow temperature for a long time. However, the preserved cells will be able to resume their normal physiological functions following recovery, if their physical structure and vitality are protected during the process and period of preservation. The methods for preserving living cells at ultralow temperature essentially employ these principles and the process is known as cryopreservation. It is the technique for preserving living cells or tissues at ultralow temperature, typically in liquid nitrogen (−196°C), at genetically and physiologically stabilized state.

Species	Oocyte	Embryo
Cow	1992 [3]	1973 [4]
Rabbit	1989 [5, 6]	1974 [7]
Sheep	—	1976 [8]
Goat	—	1976 [9]
Horse	2002 [10]	1982 [11]
Pig	2014 [12]	1989 [13]
Buffalo	—	1993 [14]

Table 1.
First reported birth from the cryopreserved oocytes and embryos in different livestock species.

Preservation of oocytes and embryos is an integral part of the assisted reproductive technologies. It allows not only preserving the valuable female germplasm but also the rapid induction of genetic merits into population through in vitro fertilization and embryo transfer. The mammalian embryos could be cryopreserved successfully for the first time in 1972. It was shown that 50–70% of the early stage mouse embryos survived freezing to −196°C that required slow cooling and slow warming [2]. Subsequently, considerable efforts have been made until now to cryopreserve oocytes and embryos in different mammalian species including livestock (**Table 1**). The field of gamete cryobiology has undergone a tremendous advancement during the last five decades.

Cryopreservation of mammalian gamete has many potential applications. Cryobanking of oocytes and embryos derived from genetically superior animals is promising for enhancing the outcome of planned breeding programs. The technique is equally important for conserving biodiversity of endangered animal species and, valuable and genetically modified laboratory animals. It also ensures steady supply of oocytes and embryos for many downstream applications of assisted reproduction such as in vitro embryo production, embryo transfer, production of stem cells, and genetic engineering.

The underlying effects of cryopreservation on mammalian oocytes and embryos have been studied extensively by the scholars worldwide. Several methods have been demonstrated for cryopreserving oocytes and embryos in different species and some of these methods are real breakthroughs. Currently, devices and consumables required for cryopreservation are available commercially from many firms that transform the procedure into a routine practice in humans as well as in livestock. In this chapter, the fundamental aspects of oocyte and embryo cryopreservation are discussed in detail.

2. Principles of cryopreservation

The process of cryopreservation exposes the cells to very low temperatures for preserving their structural and functional entity for a long period of time. As such, the freezing of cells results in the formation of both intracellular and extracellular sharp ice crystals that damage the cellular membranes and organelles and render the cells nonviable. Further, the formation of ice crystals causes osmotic stress to the cells that result from the altered concentration of intracellular solutes. Therefore, any cryopreservation protocol fundamentally includes steps that prevent and ameliorate such damages to cells during freezing. These damages are avoided by controlling the temperature during the freezing process and by incubating cells to cryoprotective solution [15]. A rapid freezing process helps avoiding the mechanical damage caused by the piercing action of ice crystals, and the rise in intracellular solute concentration can be avoided by exposing cells to cryoprotectants [15]. Permeating cryoprotective agent (CPA) decreases ice formation by replacing the intracellular liquid [16].

Irrespective of the methods, cryopreservation of oocytes and embryos basically includes four steps (**Figure 1**). Step 1: cells are equilibrated in a CPA solution that causes water egress from the cells and their dehydration. Replacement of intracellular water with permeable CPA lowers the freezing point of the intracellular content and reduces the extent of intracellular ice crystal formation. Step 2: equilibrated cells are cooled to low temperature and then stored in liquid nitrogen (−196°C). The cells are actually frozen during this step and, depending upon the cooling methods, either small intracellular ice crystals are formed (slow cooling) or the intracellular content is transformed into glass-like state bypassing ice crystal formation (vitrification). Step 3: cryopreserved cells are recovered by thawing and warming that reverse the frozen state of the cells. Step 4: finally, the thawed and warmed cells are

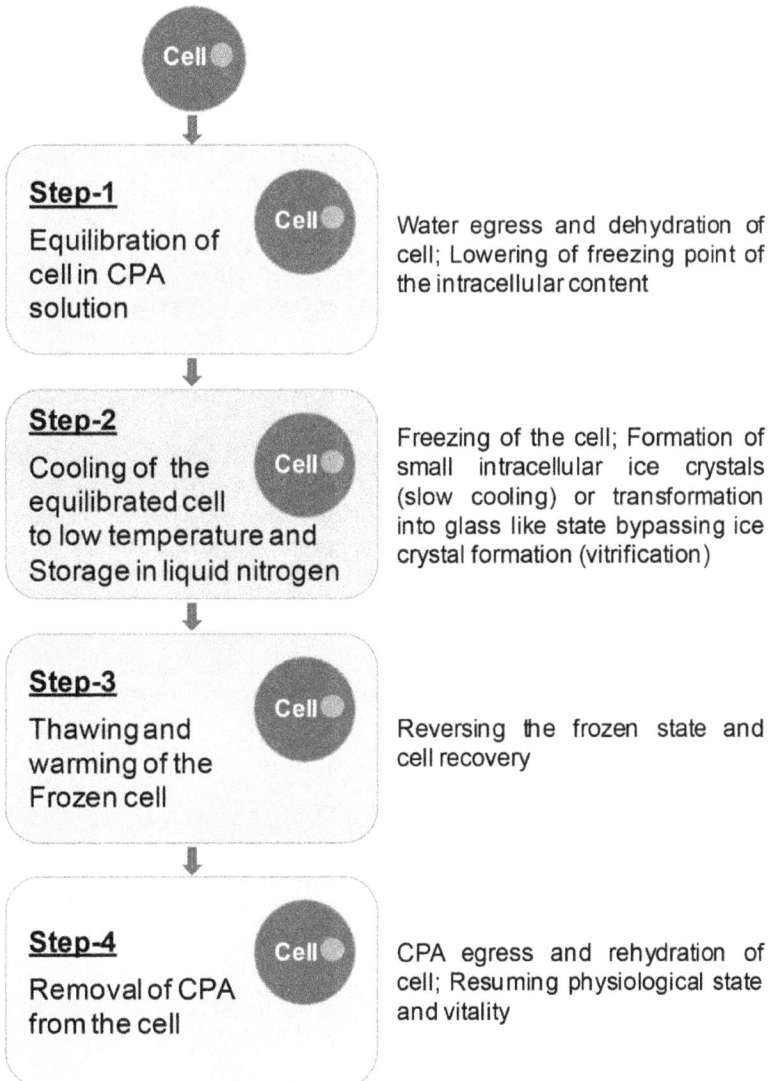

Figure 1.
Steps involved in cryopreservation of oocytes and embryos.

equilibrated in the rehydration solution that causes the replacement of intracellular CPA with water molecules. Following this step, the preserved cells regain their vitality and resume normal physiological processes.

3. Cryoprotectants

CPAs play key roles in protecting the vitality of the cryopreserved cells during their processing and storage at ultralow temperature and their subsequent recovery with normal physiological functionality. Christopher Polge and his colleagues discovered the cryoprotective capabilities of glycerol in the late 1940s that subsequently led to the successful cryopreservation of cattle and poultry spermatozoa [17]. This discovery introduced a fascinating branch of bio-physical science, the cryobiology. CPAs are water-soluble chemical substances with low level of cytotoxicity that lower the melting point of water. CPAs can be divided into two categories, membrane permeating and membrane non-permeating.

Membrane-permeating CPAs are small molecules that easily penetrate the cell membranes. During cryopreservation, these agents decrease freezing point and prevent cell damage from high electrolyte concentrations. They form linkages with the electrolyte molecules and thus act as partial substitute to water [18]. Penetrating CPAs also stabilize lipid membranes by hydrogen bonding with the membrane lipids, which is especially important under severely dehydrated conditions.

On the other hand, the non-permeating CPAs increase the viscosity of the cryopreservation solution generating osmotic gradient across the cell membrane and thus withdraw intracellular water [19]. These agents allow effective dehydration of the cells even in the presence of permeating CPAs at low concentration. Additionally, non-permeating CPAs also reduce mechanical stress that occurs during cryopreservation [20]. The list of CPAs commonly used for cryopreservation of oocytes and embryos is provided in **Table 2**.

It may be noted that no permeating CPA is completely devoid of the capability to induce cell toxicity. Therefore, the use of a single permeating CPA substantially increases the possibility of cellular toxicity to the frozen cells, because of their high concentration in the cryopreservation solution. In contrast, similar viscosity of cryopreservation solution can be achieved by using a combination of permeating CPAs along with non-permeating cryoprotective agents. In the latter case, the

Permeating cryoprotectants	Non-permeating cryoprotectants
Ethylene glycol	Glucose
Dimethyl sulfoxide	Sucrose
Propylene glycol	Trehalose
Formamide	Raffinose
Acetamide	Polyvinyl pyrrolidone
Dimethyl acetamide	Mannitol
	Ficoll
	Polyethylene glycol
	Polyvinyl alcohol
	Bovine serum albumin

Table 2.
Commonly used cryoprotectants for cryopreservation of oocytes and embryos.

concentration of a particular permeating CPA would be much lower in the solution. Therefore, it is believed that the CPA-mediated toxicity to the cells can be reduced if a combination of CPAs is used for cryopreservation.

4. Methods of cryopreservation

Fundamentally, two methods are available for cryopreserving oocytes and embryos. These are slow freezing and vitrification. The major differences between these two methods are the concentration of CPA used and the rate of cooling of sample during the preservation process (**Table 3**). However, an improved and modified version of the traditional vitrification process has been developed later that utilizes extremely high cooling rate as compared to the slow freezing or traditional vitrification procedures (**Table 3**). This improved vitrification method is known as ultrarapid vitrification.

4.1 Slow freezing

The technique of slow freezing was introduced first for cryopreserving oocytes and embryos. The technique was developed during the early 1970s [2, 21, 22] and it was considered as a gold standard for long for cryopreserving oocytes and embryos. In this technique, samples are equilibrated to a concentration gradient of

Particulars	Methods		
	Slow freezing	**Conventional vitrification**	**Ultrarapid vitrification**
Concentration of cryoprotectants	Low, 1–2 M	High, 5–7 M	Moderate, 3.5–5.5 M
Sample volume	>100 μl	50–100 μl	≤5 μl
Cooling procedure	Slow and controlled cooling with the help of a programmable freezing machine	No freezing machine is required; samples are directly plunged into liquid nitrogen	No freezing machine is required; samples are directly plunged into liquid nitrogen or placed onto a surface cooled to the temperature of liquid nitrogen
Sample processing time	Extended, 2–3 h	Short, <10 min	Short, <10 min
Formation of ice crystal	Yes	No	No
Likely osmotic injury	Low	High	Moderate
Likely CPA-mediated toxic injury	Low	High	Moderate
Likely chilling injury	High	Low	Low
Sample container	Conventional 0.25-ml straw	Conventional 0.25-ml straw	Container less or specialized container other than conventional straw
Status of system	Closed	Closed	Closed or open
Requirement of skill	Easy to perform	Difficult to perform	Difficult to perform

Table 3.
Comparison among the methods of slow freezing, vitrification, and ultrarapid vitrification.

CPAs (1–2 M final concentration) to minimize chemical and osmotic toxicity and to maintain a balance between the factors that influence cell damage [23]. Following equilibration, the samples are loaded into straws and cooled at 1–2°C/min to −5 to −7°C and then seeded to initiate extracellular freezing. Thereafter, the samples are cooled slowly at 0.3–1°C/min until they attain the temperature anywhere between −30 and −70°C [24, 25] and finally the samples are plunged into liquid nitrogen for storage. The controlled cooling of samples is achieved with the help of a programmable freezing machine. During controlled cooling, exchange of water molecules takes place between the extracellular and intracellular fluids without adverse osmotic effects [26]. Nevertheless, the extracellular and intracellular water precipitate and form ice crystals during slow cooling [27].

4.2 Conventional vitrification

Vitrification is an alternative to the slow freezing technique. This method allows solidification of the cell and the extracellular milieu into a glass-like state bypassing the formation of ice crystals. The first successful event of vitrification was reported in 1985 [16], and ice-free cryopreservation of mouse embryos at −196°C was demonstrated. Thereafter, enormous efforts have been made worldwide to utilize and improve this technique for cryopreserving oocytes and embryos in different species. Vitrification is now considered to be a proven method of cryopreservation. In this technique, cells are incubated in CPA solutions from low to high viscosity, loaded into straw, and directly plunged into liquid nitrogen. The process requires much greater cooling rate during freezing and high concentrations of CPA as compared to slow freezing. There are three important factors that ensure the vitrification process:

Cryopreservation technique	Cooling rate	Warming rate
Slow freezing	1–2°C/min until −5 to −7°C followed by 0.3–1°C/min until −30 to −70°C and then plunging sample into liquid nitrogen	250–600°C/min
Conventional vitrification	2000–2500°C/min	250–600°C/min
Ultrarapid vitrification		
Open pulled straw	20,000°C/min	20,000°C/min
Closed pulled straw	8100°C/min	—
Electron microscopic grid	180,000°C/min	—
Cryoloop	15,000°C/min	45,000°C/min
Hemi-straw	>20,000°C/min	—
Cryotop	23,000°C/min	42,000°C/min
CryoTip	12,000°C/min	24,000°C/min
Quartz micro-capillary	250,000°C/min	—
Glass capillary	12,000°C/min	62,000°C/min

Table 4.
Cooling and warming rates of different vitrification methods.

(1) viscosity of the CPA solution; (2) cooling rate; and (3) sample volume. Thus, a delicate balance must be maintained among these factors to achieve successful vitrification [1]. Vitrification can be achieved with a CPA concentration of 5–7 M and a cooling rate of approximately 2500°C/min [28]. A major advantage of vitrification is the low risk of freezing injury, thereby ensuring a sufficiently high cell survival rate.

4.3 Ultrarapid vitrification

Ultrarapid vitrification is the modified and improved version of the conventional vitrification procedure. The concept of ultrarapid cooling for cryopreserving oocytes and embryos was introduced by Vajta and his co-workers with their invention of the open pulled straw [29, 30]. The viscosity of the vitrification medium and cooling rate are inversely related. Thus, a medium containing lesser concentration of cryoprotectants and other additives can be vitrified efficiently at higher cooling rate. Theoretically, vitrification can be achieved with a 1.5 M concentration of any cryoprotectant, providing a cooling rate of 15,000°C/min is employed [28]. Ultrarapid vitrification technique employs extremely high cooling and warming rates as compared to the slow freezing or conventional vitrification methods (**Table 4**). It allows vitrification of relatively low concentration of CPA solution using extremely high cooling rate and thus reduces the CPA-mediated toxicity and osmotic stress to the vitrified cells. The ultrarapid cooling rate is achieved by reducing the effective volume of the solution to be vitrified. At present, this method is considered to be the most superior, and high post freeze-thaw survival of oocytes and embryos has been demonstrated using this method in different mammalian species.

5. Cryoinjury

Oocytes and embryos are susceptible to different types of injuries following cryopreservation, which are collectively known as cryoinjuries. The extent of cryoinjuries to the frozen oocytes and embryos depends on many factors. The major factors are the type of CPA and freezing technique used for cryopreservation and the physiological quality, chilling sensitivity, plasma membrane permeability, tolerance for osmotic stress, developmental stage, and species of the oocytes and embryos [26, 31]. One of the primary focuses during the development of cryopreservation protocols is to minimize the possibilities of cryoinjuries to the preserved oocytes and embryos following freeze-thawing. The different types of cryoinjuries that oocyte and embryos are exposed to during the cryopreservation process are described below.

5.1 Chilling injury

Chilling injuries refer to the irreversible changes that occur to the intracellular lipid droplets, lipid-containing membranes, and the cytoskeleton, during the cooling phase between +15 and −5°C [32]. Such injuries are commonly associated with the slow freezing technique. In contrast, the vitrification method substantially reduces the chances of chilling injuries to the frozen oocytes and embryos as they are exposed very briefly to the dangerous temperature zone due to high cooling rate [33]. Therefore, effective cryopreservation of porcine embryos containing extremely large amounts of chill-sensitive lipid droplets can be achieved only through vitrification [34]. Similarly, high survivability of cryopreserved oocytes of various other species such as cattle, sheep, and horse that are sensitive to chilling could be achieved through vitrification [35].

5.2 Formation of ice crystal

The formation of ice crystals during cryopreservation is the major source of cryoinjury [36]. The slow freezing method induces ice crystal formation in the aqueous phase surrounding cells as well as inside the cells including the cytoplasm and nucleus at the temperature zone between -5 and $-80°C$. In contrast, high CPA concentration and rapid cooling rate of vitrification method allow solidification of intracellular and extracellular water into a glass-like state bypassing the formation of ice crystals.

5.3 Fracture damage

Fracture damages to the zona pellucida and blastomeres of oocytes and embryos are commonly observed following cryopreservation. Such damages usually occur during freezing because of the mechanical effect of the solidified solution at the temperature zone between -50 and $-150°C$ [37].

5.4 Formation of multiple asters

Aster formation is a newly discovered form of cryoinjury. It is frequently observed in the vitrified-warmed and fertilized oocytes [38]. This cryoinjury is likely accountable for the loss of ooplasmic function responsible for normal micro-tubule assembly. The exposure of oocytes to high CPA concentration and ultrarapid cooling during vitrification leads to the formation of multiple asters near the male pronucleus. The migration and development of pronuclei are disrupted by the asters resulting in delayed first cleavage and reduced blastocyst development [38].

5.5 Osmotic stress

During the pre-freezing stage of cryopreservation, incubation of cells with high osmolar cryoprotectant solution causes cell shrinkage due to the outward movement of intracellular water in response to the difference in osmotic pressure between intracellular and extracellular solutions. Similarly, at the stage of thawing and CPA removal, the movement of water molecules occurs at the reverse direction that causes cell swelling. These phenomena are known as osmotic stress. The frozen cells are more permeable to water than cryoprotectants as compared to their fresh counterpart [39]. Therefore, the cryopreserved cells are more susceptible to osmotic stress as compared to the non-cryopreserved cells. The vitrification method employs considerably high concentration of CPAs and therefore induces greater osmotic stress as compared to the slow freezing technique. It may be noted that the required CPA concentration for vitrification is inversely related with the cooling rate. Therefore, a practical approach to reduce osmotic stress and CPA-mediated cell toxicity during vitrification is to increase the cooling rate and simultaneously reduce the concentration of CPAs.

6. Deleterious effects of cryopreservation

Cryopreservation of oocytes and embryos is associated with several deleterious consequences that in turn exert negative effects on their post freeze-thaw survivability and development.

Osmotic shock during cryopreservation and thawing may result in excessive shrinkage or swelling of cells that can damage the cellular cytoskeleton and in turn the post freeze-thaw survivability and developmental ability of the cryopreserved cells. Similarly, the formation of intracellular ice crystals during freezing may damage the cellular cytoskeleton and cell organelles.

Mitochondria are the most abundant organelles in mammalian oocytes and embryos and they are the sole source of energy production. Mitochondrial dysfunction or abnormalities are critical for the development of oocytes and embryos. A reduction in the production of ATP by mitochondria is associated with the developmental failure of oocytes and embryos [40]. Cryopreservation may contribute to mitochondrial dysfunction, mitochondrial swelling [41, 42], abnormally shaped mitochondria, rupture of mitochondrial membranes [43, 44], and reduced cellular ATP content that might contribute to poor oocyte and embryo development following freeze-thawing [45, 46].

It is evident that cryopreservation incurs negative effect on the expression of genes associated with oxidative stress, apoptosis, cell developmental process, and sperm-oocyte interaction [31, 47]. Such alteration in gene expression is one of the contributory factors of cryopreservation toward poor developmental ability of cryopreserved oocytes and embryos.

Cryopreservation can be a potential cause of physical damage to DNA. The fragmentation of DNA increases in mouse and bovine oocytes following vitrification [48, 49]. It is suggested that slow freezing as well as vitrification affect the DNA integrity in embryos [50]. Further, cryoprotectants such as ethylene glycol and propanediol increase DNA fragmentation in porcine embryos, even without a cycle of freezing and thawing [51].

Cryopreservation may induce epigenetic changes in the genome of cryopreserved oocyte and embryos. Vitrification reduces or increases gene methylation in bovine and mouse oocytes and embryos [52–55]. Further, several reports indicate that vitrification significantly alters acetylation patterns in oocytes [56, 57]. It is suggested that the aberrant epigenetic modifications in response to cryopreservation are at least partially responsible for the reduced developmental competence of frozen oocytes and embryos [31].

7. Difficulties associated with oocyte cryopreservation

The cryopreservation of oocyte is more challenging than that of the embryos. As compared to an embryo, an oocyte has to maintain integrity of many of its unique structural features following freeze-thawing to undergo fertilization and further development. Oocyte being a single cell is more vulnerable to the steps of cryopreservation as compared to a multi-cellular preimplantation embryo. The larger volume of oocyte decreases the surface-to-volume ratio that makes it very sensitive to chilling and intracellular ice formation [58, 59]. The plasma membrane of matured oocytes has a low permeability coefficient, thus making the movement of cryoprotectants and water slower [60].

In oocytes, the meiotic spindles play crucial roles in meiotic progression as well as chromosomal alignment and segregation [61]. Severe disorganization or disappearance of meiotic spindles is evident following slow freezing as well as vitrification with a more deleterious effect of the slow freezing procedure [31]. Cryopreservation exerts a negative influence on microfilament functions in oocytes that in turn can lead to abnormal distributions of mitochondria in the oolemma [6, 62, 63]. This consequently may result in reduced meiotic competence and fertilization ability of oocytes and developmental failure of early stage embryos.

During cryopreservation, CPA causes transient increase in the intracellular concentration of calcium in oocytes [64] that triggers exocytosis of cortical granule [65] resulting in hardening of zona pellucida and in turn compromised sperm penetration and fertilization [66].

8. Future perspectives

The procedures of oocyte and embryo cryopreservation have evolved significantly since it was demonstrated for the first time five decades ago. Nevertheless, the success of oocyte cryopreservation is considerably poor as compared to that of the embryos at late developmental stage, even following the ultrarapid vitrification, which is considered as the best technique at present. Therefore, currently, the most important challenge in this field is to develop standardized protocols for effective cryopreservation of oocytes and early stage embryos. The theoretical target of success of such protocols should be comparable with that of their non-cryopreserved counterpart. It is evident from the current state of knowledge that the ability of oocytes and embryos to withstand cryopreservation process varies among the different species. It appears impossible to develop a single standardized protocol for all species. Therefore, future efforts should focus on developing species-specific optimized protocols for oocyte and embryo cryopreservation. Further, it will be fascinating to observe future efforts for the development of automated devices for oocyte and embryo vitrification. The implementation of an efficient and automated ultrarapid vitrification system for routine use in livestock can revolutionize the field worldwide. Conclusively, the most prominent future targets of cryopreservation are expected to focus on the development of protocols that would maintain as much as possible the structural and functional integrities of oocytes and embryos following freeze-thawing. The outcome of such protocols should be reproducible as well across the laboratories worldwide. Realization of such targets would definitely lead to the development of standardized and optimized methods for oocyte and embryo cryopreservation for routine use in livestock.

9. Conclusions

Cryopreservation is the technique to preserve living cells at ultralow temperature, typically in liquid nitrogen (−196°C). Cryopreservation of oocytes and embryos is extremely important for propagation and conservation of genetically superior germplasm. Any cryopreservation protocol basically includes three major steps such as equilibration of cells to concentrated solution of cryoprotective agent, cooling and storage of cells to ultralow temperature, and recovery of frozen cells following thawing and warming. Cryoprotective agents protect vitality of the cryopreserved cells during processing and storage at ultralow temperature. Basically, there are two fundamental methods for cryopreserving oocytes and embryos, slow freezing and vitrification. The slow freezing method involves cooling of the samples slowly at controlled rate and formation of intracellular and extracellular ice crystals. In contrast, the conventional vitrification method involves rapid cooling of the samples and solidification of the cells including extracellular milieu into a glass-like state bypassing ice crystal formation. Ultrarapid vitrification is the modified and improved version of the conventional vitrification procedure that involves extremely high cooling and warming rates. Currently, ultrarapid vitrification is considered to be the more superior method than slow freezing or conventional vitrification. It is evident that cryopreservation often results in different types of cryoinjuries such as chilling injury, formation of ice crystal, fracture damage, osmotic stress, and formation of multiple asters. The quantum of cryoinjuries to frozen cells depends on many factors. Cryoinjuries are responsible for poor survivability of the cryopreserved cells. The cryopreservation process is associated with several other deleterious consequences and those in turn exert negative effects on the post freeze-thaw survivability of the frozen cells. Cryopreservation of oocytes is more difficult and yields poor success because of their larger volume and unique structural features as compared to that of the embryos. The procedures of oocyte and embryo cryopreservation have evolved significantly over the past five decades. Yet, the species-specific optimized cryopreservation methods with reproducible results are not available currently, especially for the oocytes and early stage embryos.

Conflict of interest

None.

Author details

Arindam Dhali*, Atul P. Kolte, Ashish Mishra, Sudhir C. Roy
and Raghavendra Bhatta
ICAR-National Institute of Animal Nutrition and Physiology, Bengaluru, India

*Address all correspondence to: dhali72@gmail.com

IntechOpen

References

[1] Jang TH, Parka SC, Yanga JH, Kima JY, Seoka JH, Parka US, et al. Cryopreservation and its clinical applications. Integrative Medicine Research. 2017;**6**:12-18. DOI: 10.1016/j.imr.2016.12.001

[2] Whittingham DG, Leibo SP, Mazur P. Survival of mouse embryos frozen to −196 degrees and −269 degrees C. Science. 1972;**178**:411-414. DOI: 10.1126/science.178.4059.411

[3] Fuku E, Kojima T, Shioya Y, Marcus GJ, Downey BR. In vitro fertilization and development of frozen-thawed bovine oocytes. Cryobiology. 1992;**29**:485-492. DOI: 10.1016/0011-2240(92)90051-3

[4] Wilmut I, Rowson LEA. Experiments in the low temperature preservation of cow embryos. The Veterinary Record. 1973;**92**:686-690. DOI: 10.1136/vr.92.26.686

[5] Al-Hasani S, Krisch J, Diedrich K, Blanke S, van der Ven H, Krebs D. Successful embryo transfer of cryopreserved and in-vitro fertilized rabbit oocytes. Human Reproduction. 1989;**4**:77-79. DOI: 10.1093/oxfordjournals.humrep.a136849

[6] Vincent C, Garnier V, Heyman Y, Renard JP. Solvent effects on cytoskeletal organization and in vivo survival after freezing of rabbit oocytes. Journal of Reproduction and Fertility. 1989;**87**:809-820. DOI: 10.1530/jrf.0.0870809

[7] Bank H, Maurer RR. Survival of frozen rabbit embryos. Experimental Cell Research. 1974;**89**:188-196. DOI: 10.1016/0014-4827(74)90201-8

[8] Willadsen SM, Polge C, Rowson LE, Moor RM. Deep freezing of sheep embryos. Journal of Reproduction and Fertility. 1976;**46**:151-154. DOI: 10.1530/jrf.0.0460151

[9] Bilton RJ, Moore RW. In vitro culture, storage, and transfer of goat embryos. Australian Journal of Biological Sciences. 1976;**29**:125-129. DOI: 10.1071/BI9760125

[10] Maclellan LJ, Carnevale EM, Coutinho da Silva MA, Scoggin CF, Bruemmer JE, Squires EL. Pregnancies from vitrified equine oocytes collected from superstimulated and non-stimulated mares. Theriogenology. 2002;**58**:911-919. DOI: 10.1016/S0093-691X(02)00920-2

[11] Yamamoto YN, Oguri N, Tsutsumi Y, Hachinohe Y. Experiments in the freezing and storage of equine embryos. Journal of Reproduction and Fertility. 1982;**32**:399-403

[12] Somfai T, Yoshiok K, Tanihara F, Kaneko H, Noguchi J, Kashiwazaki N, et al. Generation of live piglets from cryopreserved oocytes for the first time using a defined system for in vitro embryo production. PLoS One. 2014;**9**:e97731. DOI: 10.1371/journal.pone.0097731

[13] Hayashi S, Kobayashi K, Mizuno J, Saitoh K, Hirano S. Birth of piglets from frozen embryos. The Veterinary Record. 1989;**125**:43-44. DOI: 10.1136/vr.125.2.43

[14] Kasiraj R, Misra AK, Mutha Rao M, Jaiswal RS, Rangareddi NS. Successful culmination of pregnancy and live birth following the transfer of frozen–thawed buffalo embryos. Theriogenology. 1993;**39**:1187-1192. DOI: 10.1016/0093-691X(93)90016-X

[15] Mandawala AA, Harvey SC, Roy TK, Fowler KE. Cryopreservation of animal oocytes and embryos: Current progress and future prospects. Theriogenology. 2016;**86**:1637-1644. DOI: 10.1016/j.theriogenology.2016.07.018

[16] Rall WF, Fahy GM. Ice-free cryopreservation of mouse embryos at −196°C by vitrification. Nature. 1985;**313**:573-575. DOI: 10.1038/313573a0

[17] Polge C, Smith AU, Parkes AS. Revival of spermatozoa after vitrification and dehydration at low temperatures. Nature. 1949;**164**:666. DOI: 10.1038/164666a0

[18] Rall WF, Reid DS, Polge C. Analysis of slow-warming injury of mouse embryos by cryomicroscopical and physiocheminal methods. Cryobiology. 1984;**21**:106-121. DOI: 10.1016/0011-2240(84)90027-0

[19] Orief Y, Schultze-Mosgau A, Dafopoulos K, Al-Hasani S. Vitrification: Will it replace the conventional gamete cryopreservation techniques? Middle East Fertility Society Journal. 2005;**10**:171-184

[20] Dumoulin JC, Janssen JMB, Pieters MH, Enginsu ME, Geraedts JP, Evers JL. The protective effects of polymers in the cryopreservation of human and mouse zonae pellucidae and embryos. Fertility and Sterility. 1994;**62**:793-798. DOI: 10.1016/S0015-0282(16)57006-X

[21] Whittingham DG. Survival of mouse embryos after freezing and thawing. Nature. 1971;**233**:125-126. DOI: 10.1038/233125a0

[22] Wilmut I. The effect of cooling rate, warming rate, cryoprotective agent and stage of development of survival of mouse embryos during freezing and thawing. Life Sciences. 1972;**11**:1071-1079. DOI: 10.1016/0024-3205(72)90215-9

[23] Pereira RM, Marques C. Animal oocyte and embryo cryopreservation. Cell and Tissue Banking. 2008;**9**:267-277. DOI: 10.1007/s10561-008-9075-2

[24] Saragusty J, Arav A. Current progress in oocyte and embryo

cryopreservation by slow freezing and vitrification. Reproduction. 2011;**141**: 1-19. DOI: 10.1530/REP-10-0236

[25] Rienzi L, Gracia C, Maggiulli R, LaBarbera AR, Kaser DJ, Ubaldi FM, et al. Oocyte, embryo and blastocyst cryopreservation in ART: Systematic review and meta-analysis comparing slow-freezing versus vitrification to produce evidence for the development of global guidance. Human Reproduction Update. 2017;**23**:139-155. DOI: 10.1093/humupd/dmw038

[26] Vajta G, Kuwayama M. Improving cryopreservation systems. Theriogenology. 2006;**65**:236-244. DOI: 10.1016/j.theriogenology.2005.09.026

[27] Prentice JR, Anzar M. Cryopreservation of mammalian oocyte for conservation of animal genetics. Veterinary Medicine International. 2011;**2011**:146405. DOI: 10.4061/2011/146405

[28] Palasz AT, Mapletoft RJ. Cryopreservation of mammalian embryos and oocytes: Recent advances. Biotechnology Advances. 1996;**14**:127-149. DOI: 10.1016/0734-9750(96)00005-5

[29] Vajta G, Booth PJ, Holm P, Greve T, Callesen H. Successful vitrification of early stage bovine in vitro produced embryos with the open pulled straw (OPS) method. Cryo-Letters. 1997;**18**:191-195

[30] Vajta G, Holm P, Kuwayama M, Booth PJ, Jacobsen H, Greve T, et al. Open pulled straw (OPS) vitrification: A new way to reduce cryoinjuries of bovine ova and embryos. Molecular Reproduction and Development. 1998;**51**:53-58. DOI: 10.1002/(SICI)1098-2795(199809)51

[31] Moussa M, Shu J, Zhang X, Zeng F. Cryopreservation of mammalian oocytes and embryos: Current problems

and future perspectives. Science China. Life Sciences. 2014;**57**:903-914. DOI: 10.1007/s11427-014-4689-z

[32] Vajta G. Vitrification of the oocytes and embryos of domestic animals. Animal Reproduction Science. 2000;**60-61**:357-364. DOI: 10.1016/S0378-4320(00)00097-X

[33] Rall W. Factors affecting the survival of mouse embryos cryopreserved by vitrification. Cryobiology. 1987;**24**:387-402. DOI: 10.1016/0011-2240(87)90042-3

[34] Berthelot F, Martinat-Botté F, Perreau C, Terqui M. Birth of piglets after OPS vitrification and transfer of compacted morula stage embryos with intact zona pellucida. Reproduction, Nutrition, Development. 2001;**41**:267-272. DOI: 10.1051/rnd:2001129

[35] Ledda S, Bogliolo L, Succu S, Ariu F, Bebbere D, Leoni GG, et al. Oocyte cryopreservation: Oocyte assessment and strategies for improving survival. Reproduction, Fertility, and Development. 2007;**19**:13-23. DOI: 10.1071/RD06126

[36] Paynter SJ. A rational approach to oocyte cryopreservation. Reproductive Biomedicine Online. 2005;**10**:578-586. DOI: 10.1016/S1472-6483(10)61664-1

[37] Rall W, Meyer T. Zona fracture damage and its avoidance during the cryopreservation of mammalian embryos. Theriogenology. 1989;**31**:683-692. DOI: 10.1016/0093-691X(89)90251-3

[38] Hara H, Hwang IS, Kagawa N, Kuwayama M, Hirabayashi M, Hochi S. High incidence of multiple aster formation in vitrified-warmed bovine oocytes after in vitro fertilization. Theriogenology. 2012;**77**:908-915. DOI: 10.1016/j.theriogenology.2011.09.018

[39] Pedro PB, Zhu SE, Makino N. Effects of hypotonic stress on the survival of mouse oocytes and embryos at various stages. Cryobiology. 1997;**35**:150-158. DOI: 10.1006/cryo.1997.2034

[40] Brevini TA, Vassena R, Francisci C, Gandolfi F. Role of adenosine triphosphate, active mitochondria, and microtubules in the acquisition of developmental competence of parthenogenetically activated pig oocytes. Biology of Reproduction. 2005;**72**:1218-1223. DOI: 10.1095/biolreprod.104.038141

[41] Valojerdi MR, Salehnia M. Developmental potential and ultrastructural injuries of metaphase II (MII) mouse oocytes after slow freezing or vitrification. Journal of Assisted Reproduction and Genetics. 2005;**22**:119-127. DOI: 10.1007/s10815-005-4876-8

[42] Hochi S, Kozawa M, Fujimoto T, Hondo E, Yamada J, Oguri N. In vitro maturation and transmission electron microscopic observation of horse oocytes after vitrification. Cryobiology. 1996;**33**:300-310. DOI: 10.1006/cryo.1996.0030

[43] Wu C, Rui R, Dai J, Zhang C, Ju S, Xie B, et al. Effects of cryopreservation on the developmental competence, ultrastructure and cytoskeletal structure of porcine oocytes. Molecular Reproduction and Development. 2006;**73**:1454-1462. DOI: 10.1002/mrd.20579

[44] Turathum B, Saikhun K, Sangsuwan P, Kitiyanant Y. Effects of vitrification on nuclear maturation, ultrastructural changes and gene expression of canine oocytes. Reproductive Biology and Endocrinology. 2010;**8**:70. DOI: 10.1186/1477-7827-8-70

[45] Manipalviratn S, Tong ZB, Stegmann B, Widra E, Carter J, DeCherney A. Effect of vitrification and thawing on human oocyte ATP

concentration. Fertility and Sterility. 2011;**95**:1839-1841. DOI: 10.1016/j.fertnstert.2010.10.040

[46] Zhao XM, Du WH, Wang D, Hao HS, Liu Y, Qin T, et al. Effect of cyclosporine pretreatment on mitochondrial function in vitrified bovine mature oocytes. Fertility and Sterility. 2011;**95**:2786-2788. DOI: 10.1016/j.fertnstert.2011.04.089

[47] Lin C, Tsai S. The effect of cryopreservation on DNA damage, gene expression and protein abundance in vertebrate. Italian Journal of Animal Science. 2012;**11**:e21. DOI: 10.4081/ijas.2012.e21

[48] Huang JY, Chen HY, Park JY, Tan SL, Chian RC. Comparison of spindle and chromosome configuration in in vitro- and in vivo-matured mouse oocytes after vitrification. Fertility and Sterility. 2008;**90**:1424-1432. DOI: 10.1016/j.fertnstert.2007.07.1335

[49] Stachowiak EM, Papis K, Kruszewski M, Iwanen'ko T, Bartłomiejczyk T, Modlin'ski JA. Comparison of the level(s) of DNA damage using Comet assay in bovine oocytes subjected to selected vitrification methods. Reproduction in Domestic Animals. 2009;**44**:653-658. DOI: 10.1111/j.1439-0531.2007.01042.x

[50] Kader A, Agarwal A, Abdelrazik H, Sharma RK, Ahmady A, Falcone T. Evaluation of post-thaw DNA integrity of mouse blastocysts after ultrarapid and slow freezing. Fertility and Sterility. 2009;**91**:2087-2094. DOI: 10.1016/j.fertnstert.2008.04.049

[51] Rajaei F, Karja NW, Agung B, Wongsrikeao P, Taniguchi M, Murakami M, et al. Analysis of DNA fragmentation of porcine embryos exposed to cryoprotectants. Reproduction in Domestic Animals. 2005;**40**:429-432. DOI: 10.1111/j.1439-0531.2005.00585.x

[52] Zhao XM, Ren JJ, Du WH, Hao HS, Wang D, Liu Y, et al. Effect of 5-aza-2'-deoxycytidine on methylation of the putative imprinted control region of H19 during the in vitro development of vitrified bovine two-cell embryos. Fertility and Sterility. 2012;**98**:222-227. DOI: 10.1016/j.fertnstert.2012.04.014

[53] Zhao XM, Du WH, Hao HS, Wang D, Qin T, Liu Y, et al. Effect of vitrification on promoter methylation and the expression of pluripotency and differentiation genes in mouse blastocysts. Molecular Reproduction and Development. 2012;**79**:445-450. DOI: 10.1002/mrd.22052

[54] Milroy C, Liu L, Hammoud S, Hammoud A, Peterson CM, Carrell DT. Differential methylation of pluripotency gene promoters in in vitro matured and vitrified, in vivo-matured mouse oocytes. Fertility and Sterility. 2011;**95**:2094-2099. DOI: 10.1016/j.fertnstert.2011.02.011

[55] Yan LY, Yan J, Qiao J, Zhao PL, Liu P. Effects of oocyte vitrification on histone modifications. Reproduction, Fertility, and Development. 2010;**22**:920-925. DOI: 10.1071/RD09312

[56] Suo L, Meng Q, Pei Y, Fu X, Wang Y, Bunch TD, et al. Effect of cryopreservation on acetylation patterns of lysine 12 of histone H4 (acH4K12) in mouse oocytes and zygotes. Journal of Assisted Reproduction and Genetics. 2010;**27**:735-741. DOI: 10.1007/s10815-010-9469-5

[57] Spinaci M, Vallorani C, Bucci D, Tamanini C, Porcu E, Galeati G. Vitrification of pig oocytes induces changes in histone H4 acetylation and histone H3 lysine 9 methylation (H3K9). Veterinary Research Communications. 2012;**36**:165-171. DOI: 10.1007/s11259-012-9527-9

[58] Arav A, Zeron Y, Leslie SB, Behboodi E, Anderson GB, Crowe

JH. Phase transition temperature and chilling sensitivity of bovine oocytes. Cryobiology. 1996;**33**:589-599. DOI: 10.1006/cryo.1996.0062

[59] Zeron Y, Pearl M, Borochov A, Arav A. Kinetic and temporal factors influence chilling injury to germinal vesicle and mature bovine oocytes. Cryobiology. 1999;**38**:35-42. DOI: 10.1006/cryo.1998.2139

[60] Ruffing NA, Steponkus PL, Pitt RE, Parks JE. Osmotic behavior, hydraulic conductivity, and incidence of intracellular ice formation in bovine oocytes at different developmental stages. Cryobiology. 1993;**30**:562-580. DOI: 10.1006/cryo.1993.1059

[61] Schatten G, Simerly C, Schatten H. Microtubule configurations during fertilization, mitosis, and early development in the mouse and the requirement for egg microtubule-mediated motility during mammalian fertilization. Proceedings of the National Academy of Sciences of the United States of America. 1985;**82**:4152-4156. DOI: 10.1073/pnas.82.12.4152

[62] Zander-Fox D, Cashman KS, Lane M. The presence of 1 mM glycine in vitrification solutions protects oocyte mitochondrial homeostasis and improves blastocyst development. Journal of Assisted Reproduction and Genetics. 2013;**30**:107-116. DOI: 10.1007/s10815-012-9898-4

[63] Nagai S, Mabuchi T, Hirata S, Shoda T, Kasai T, Yokota S, et al. Correlation of abnormal mitochondrial distribution in mouse oocytes with reduced developmental competence. The Tohoku Journal of Experimental Medicine. 2006;**210**:137-144. DOI: 10.1620/tjem.210.137

[64] Larman MG, Sheehan CB, Gardner DK. Calcium-free vitrification reduces cryoprotectant-induced zona pellucida hardening and increases fertilization rates in mouse oocytes. Reproduction. 2006;**131**:53-61. DOI: 10.1530/rep.1.00878

[65] Kline D, Kline JT. Repetitive calcium transients and the role of calcium in exocytosis and cell cycle activation in the mouse egg. Developmental Biology. 1992;**149**:80-89. DOI: 10.1016/0012-1606(92)90265-I

[66] Pickering SJ, Braude PR, Johnson MH. Cryoprotection of human oocytes: Inappropriate exposure to DMSO reduces fertilization rates. Human Reproduction. 1991;**6**:142-143. DOI: 10.1093/oxfordjournals.humrep.a137248

Chapter 5

The Psychosocial Aspect of Infertility

Cicek Hocaoglu

Abstract

For both partners, infertility is a complex and situational crisis that is generically psychologically threatening, emotionally stressful, financially challenging, and physically painful most of the times due to diagnostic-curative operations undergone. Infertility triggers a range of physical, psychological, social, emotional, and financial effects. Although it is not a life-threatening problem, infertility is yet experienced as a stressful life event for couples or individuals due to the exalted value attributed to having a child by individuals themselves or society in general. Infertile couples are not facing a medical condition alone but coping with a number of emotional states as well. Emotions, thoughts, and beliefs of infertile couples frequently change as one consequence of infertility diagnosis. Exposed to a tremendous social pressure, infertile couples may resort to hiding the problem due to the extreme privacy of the matter. Infertility also affects marriage life adversely.

Keywords: infertility, psychological factors, infertile couple

1. Introduction

Although not classified as a life-threatening disease, infertility is a social problem affecting the individual, family, and society. Since infertility causes personal, familial, and social problems, it is a devastating therefore serious health problem [1, 2]. An abundance of studies have evidenced the physical, psychological, ethical, sociocultural, emotional, and financial effects of infertility. Infertile couples or individuals frequently demonstrate signs of stress, anxiety, depression, financial hardships, guilt feeling, fear, loss of social status, despondence, and social labeling [3–7]. Yet a good number of infertile couples or individuals choose to hide the problem and avoid sharing fertility problem with their families and relatives, which then leave them unsupported. In the course of time, avoidance may result in social isolation [2, 8]. As regards this matter, healthcare personnel could also fail in correctly evaluating psychological state of infertile individual or couples, or correctly diagnose psychiatric indicators and disorders. That failure could adversely affect couples' life quality and infertility treatment. In this part of study, we have systemically reviewed our latest knowledge on the psychological manifestation of infertility.

2. Infertility and reproduction

Reproduction and continuing the lineage are among the most innate and important instincts of all living beings. For both partners, infertility is a complex and situational crisis that is usually psychologically threatening, emotionally stressful, financially challenging, and physically painful most of the times due to diagnostic-curative operations undergone. The condition impacts 10–15% of couples at their reproductive age [2–7]. The incidence of infertility and etiology differ in different societies. Approximately 8–10% of couples in developed countries and 15–20% of developing countries have infertility [4]. Fertility is a vital function of adult development. If this need is unmet, as seen among infertile couples, there is a negative impact on their future plans, self-image, self-respect, marriage life, and sexual life. It is also feasible to see loss of physical and sexual privacy among such couples [9, 10].

3. Psychological factors as one reason of infertility

It was detected that causes of infertility are widely ranged for men and women. The causal factors of infertility are not limited with medical factors but extend to psychological factors too [11]. Emotional drivers of infertility for women can be listed as tubal spasm, anovulation, rapidly throwing seminal sperms, and vaginismus. Added to that, another infertility factor related to women is unintentionally avoiding sexual intercourse while ovulating. There are a number of psychological commonalities among infertile women. Although most women seem to dearly want to get pregnant and express their desire verbally, deep down they may hide negative views and fear toward pregnancy. These fears may originate from pregnancy, delivery, or motherhood. Among some of the potential underlying causes with psychogenic roots are also fear of having a bad body shape due to pregnancy, fear of losing her life or the baby during delivery, or fear of failing as a good mother. Studies revealed that if women were encouraged to express such emotions, a more affectionate and unrestricted bond could be developed among partners, which then could lead to pregnancy [12–14]. Among men, impotence in erection and ejaculation are root causes of psychological infertility. Besides, as is the case for women, men can also avoid coitus unintentionally. Male impotence may exist from birth or develop in life later. In a vast majority of men, it is also possible to experience temporary impotence in any stage of life. A great part of impotence breakout could be related to psychological causes. Most of the times, past psychological traumas, nutritional disorders, childhood diseases, and overaffectionate and protectionist mothers are among the initiative factors of psychological impotence [12, 15, 16].

4. The relationship between stress and infertility

Infertility is mainly categorized as an unsolvable life crisis that threatens being a parent, which is one of the salient life objectives, putting pressure on personal resources and having a potential to resuscitate unsolved conflicts of the past years. For infertile couples, stress sources may originate from personal, societal, and marital life. It was reported that single or collective presence of these factors increased the stress level during treatment process more [17–19]. For the couples defining their infertility experience as "the most distressing life event," overcoming their current condition can only be possible by coping the stress and adapt into the current situation. Individuals diagnosed with infertility are forced to counteract a condition not solvable with the available coping strategies. In stress management, personal capacity, past experiences, and support from immediate social circle are very critical [20]. Failure to reproduce fuels both familial and environmental pressures among couples while also igniting stress and tension at home. If failure to reproduce were perceived as if it were a crime and if it forced the individual to feel like a loser in community, infertile couples would then choose to be isolated from their close circle. As spouses become more discreet toward one another, their marriage life may also be adversely altered. Another explanation for infertility-related stress among couples is the financial cost of treatment process. Since it is a long, exhausting, and also costly stage of which treatment process is uncertain, partners are likely to undergo an emotionally difficult and tense experience. Extended length of infertility and treatment is another factor related to psychiatric problems. Sociofinancially advanced couples prove to be more apt in accepting infertility and develop favorable coping methods against infertility-induced psychological problems, but the opposite holds true among sociofinancially backward couples [16, 21–23]. On the other hand, it was acknowledged that rather than financial hardships, the influencers of quitting the treatment protocol are physical and emotional burden, huge stress, and disappointment. The same study also highlighted that feeling stressful prior to IVF operation is an acceptable case. Yet stress during the actual treatment process led to adverse consequences [24]. In one study conducted across 151 female cases to investigate the effect of stress on IVF treatment, three vital findings were obtained [25]. These findings were, respectively, listed as follows. (1) Stress level in the beginning of treatment is significantly correlated with biological parameters such as collected number of oocysts, total number of fertilized oocysts, pregnancy ratios, live birth ratios, and birth weight. (2) Stress level during IVF procedure is significantly correlated with collected number of oocysts and total number of fertilized oocysts. (3) When infertile couples having least amount of stress in the beginning are compared with the ones having most amount of stress, it is detected that frequency of dead birth is 93% lower. Stress-lowering interventions during infertility treatment are correlated with increased ratios of pregnancy. Among women with adequate level of active-effective defense mechanism and emotional self-expression, there is higher success of infertility treatment compared to women not having these traits [25]. It is reported that unpredictability, negativity, uncontrollability, and ambiguity dimensions of infertility may be perceived as stressors for individuals. The application of stress and coping theories to infertility; in which situations infertility is perceived as more stressful, what is the factors that facilitate and complicate adaptation of individual and couples diagnosed with infertility would assist in better understanding which therapeutic interventions are more beneficial for reducing stress.

5. Psychological effects of infertility on couples

When a married couple fails to reproduce despite desiring to have a baby, they feel like not fulfilling the role of "being family." Failure to accomplish reproduction function leads the couples to feel like a loser and idler. By negatively affecting social life, mood, marriage life, sexual life, future plans, self-respect, body image, and life quality of couples, infertility then turns into a complex life crisis [2, 7, 27]. For the couples, the common emotions for not having a baby are frustration and missing mother-father roles valued in society. For a woman, childlessness is associated with infertility (functional disorder), loss of control (my body rebelling against my will), psychological void (unfulfilled maternal instinct), feeling outcast from female community, feeling worthless, loneliness (lack of emotional support of the child), absence of social security (nobody to look after them in old age), unmet social role (mother, pregnant woman, postpartum period, mother-in-law), and lower self-esteem [2, 27]. For a man, childlessness is associated with failure to impregnate a woman (weak functioning of manhood), psychological void (unfulfilled paternal instinct), loneliness (in old age), failure to continue the lineage, unmet social role (father, father-in-law), and diminished social security [2, 27].

6. Reactions of couples against infertility

Despite the existence of personal differences regarding the reactions of individuals against infertility, studies also indicated a number of commonalities [2]. The ubiquitous emotion experienced by infertility-diagnosed individuals is misery. Personal reactions against infertility are confusion, denial, anger, negotiation (if I get pregnant then...), despondence, withdrawal, social isolation, lamenting, guilt feeling, unworthiness, frustration, and acceptance. The first stage is to feel shock, confusion, and disbelief. When the couple is diagnosed with infertility, first they feel shocked due to this sad fact and choose not to believe. Shock stage is followed by denial stage. Most of the times, couples are busy with not having an unplanned pregnancy so they are totally unprepared against the infertility scenario. Hence, outbreak of infertility problem is particularly devastating for those with high expectations and extreme confidence in overcoming any challenges in life. In order to avoid facing this bitter reality, denial is a popular tactic. Frustration experienced with the menstruation period every month is ignored by the couple, and infertility is attributed to fewness of sexual intercourses and believing that it is quite normal to get pregnant in the early months. Another stage awaiting the couples is fury and anxiety. An infertile partner is anxious with the fear of being left by the spouse; women feel themselves worthless and useless while men feel like having lost their manhood and might-power attributes of fatherhood. Reasons explaining the extremity of such emotions for women are fear of receiving many tests and protocols in her own body, anxiousness to lose the love of spouse, feeling worthless and useless, and a loss of self-confidence due to feeling depreciated manhood or womanhood. The longer waiting period and the more complexities in diagnosis and treatment can result in a heightened level of disappointment and anxiety trap. The next stage awaiting the couples is anger stage. Individuals feel resentful toward themselves, their partners, families, and social circle. Infertile couples feel to be treated unfairly and ask the question "Why us?" This question leads the couple to put the blame on past abortions or secret sexual intercourses that call for punishment. This accusation brings with itself self-directed anger or anger and hostility toward the partner. After all, infertility can be perceived as a problem threatening the continuity of one's lineage. The problem could even end up in solutions such as divorce, remarriage, or even suicide. Another stage awaiting infertile couples is the stage of loss of control. The complex and interventional nature of administered treatments and detailed questioning of couple's sexual life is perceived as a violation of their private life. Unpredictability of treatment success fuels a feeling of ambiguity toward the future. Couples think their private life is violated since administered treatments and directed questions expose their most-intimate life to outsiders. At this stage, women intentionally avoid seeing their pregnant friends and push themselves into loneliness. Another stage to be experienced by a couple diagnosed with infertility is the stage of guilt feeling. Infertile partner blames himself/herself due to the conviction that cultural motherhood-fatherhood role is denied from their partner because of their failure. Such feelings of blame and anger trap the infertile partner into despair. Partners feel themselves guilty since they blame themselves for denying their partner from the right of motherhood-fatherhood. As family and culture pressure are jointed with these emotions, they feel like being punished. They lose their interest to everyday life, they have lower motivation and enthusiasm and everything loses their former value, and they are likely to develop depression at this stage. For an infertile couple, each month with no pregnancy is perceived as if losing the child in the womb because of menstruation. Feeling of child loss brings mourning and depression. Although there is no tangible loss like in death or divorce, paradoxically, couples mourn for a baby who never existed in the first place. It is because the issue is not the loss of baby only; it means saying goodbye to dreams of ideal family and happy future. As time goes by, they develop apathy to life and feel beaten. In a different saying, mourning process results in depression [26, 27]. Healthy couples gradually enter into the stage of acceptance. Denials recede and facts supersede. By seeking alternative treatment options, they reconnect with each other and their friends and follow a more amiable approach in their reactions. Then these couples accept the infeasibility of having a child through biological ways. At this junction, couples need to make difficult choices like continuing a childless marriage, getting a divorce and remarrying someone else, or adopting a child [2, 7, 8, 28]. Stages of infertility are very much like the mourning process for someone nearing death. Yet, in infertility, there is not a fatal life-threatening issue; life quality and an agreeable marriage are at stake. Besides, although in a fatal disease, individuals come closer, the opposite holds true for infertility and couples distance themselves from one another as partners and from their social circle [28–31]. The reactions given to infertility may be different from among societies. Similarly, men and women exhibit different reactions against infertility. Women express their emotions more frequently and need wider social support, whereas men share their problems less frequently. As a defense mechanism, women negatively react to infertility, while men would choose to forget and deny. This disparity prevents partners to understand each other. Then, they start not to talk about their problems and women feel like shouldering this problem on their own. When the partners fail to provide emotional support to each one, family bond is destined to weaken [8, 32, 33]. In a relevant study, it was identified that among 31% of women and 16% of men, dominant emotions were despondence, pessimism, despair; 23% of women and 16% of men felt lonesome [34]. A different study focusing on the loneliness levels of infertile women revealed that 85.4% were primer infertile, 54% were woman-borne infertile, 78.7% received no psychological support [35]. In the same study, women's loneliness scores were found to be significantly related with the variables such as being employed, education level, length of infertility, number of marriage, need for psychological support, social security status, and social support [35]. Certain studies indicated that infertility affected couples' emotional state, social, sexual life, and marriage bond, and compared to men, these effects were more intensively experienced among women [36, 37].

7. Correlation between infertility and mental disorders

A number of studies have investigated the correlation between infertility and mental indicators and disorders. A vast majority of studies show that a significant correlation existed between infertility and mental indicators. It was identified that among infertile patients, the hardest psychological challenge was anxiety, and for those couples having had a failed treatment, depression was the greatest psychological burden. In an interview conducted with 112 infertile women, it was reported that psychiatric disorder was vivid across 40% of cases. The most pervasive diagnoses were reportedly anxiety disorder (23%), major depressive disorder (17%), and dysthymic disorder (9.8%) in the infertile group in Japan [36]. These findings point out that in comparison to society at large, frequency of psychiatric disorder was higher among cases with a diagnosed infertility issue. In studies encompassing different communities, it was detected that correlation existed particularly between generalized anxiety disorder and infertility [29, 38–40]. For example, generalized anxiety disorder was associated with infertility in the 11,000-person study conducted in the American community [37]. In Japanese society, which has various cultural characteristics, the results also supported the generalized anxiety disorder [14]. Similarly, in many studies from different society, the highest prevalence of anxiety and depression as a psychiatric illness were detected in patients with infertile [35, 38–40]. Infertility is also compared with chronic physical diseases. In one study that contrasted infertility-diagnosed cases with patients diagnosed with HIV-positive, cancer, cardiac disease, or similar life-threatening chronic diseases, anxiety effect was reported to be higher among the infertile group [41]. By the same token, it was identified that compared to healthy, pregnant women, infertile women maintained higher depression rates [40, 42]. Undoubtedly, the reason for more frequent depressive indicators among women is that interventional diagnosis and infertility treatment procedures are administered on women's body. In a relevant study, it was seen that compared to control group, mood disorder was reported to be 3.4 times and generalized anxiety disorder 2.7 times more widespread in infertile patient group [40]. Among infertile patients, other common psychiatric problems are sexual function disorder, somatization disorder, dysthymia, panic disorder, obsessive compulsive disorder, and social anxiety disorder. Eating disorders such as anorexia nervosa, bulimia nervosa, and obesity were reported to be linked with infertility. In addition, alcohol and drug addiction were also reportedly widespread among infertile cases. Some studies revealed that among infertile women, there was elevated level of anger and stronger aggression, while other studies showed that anger could be turned to the self or to outside. It was highlighted that among patients undergoing infertility treatment, hormonal imbalance in hypothalamus hypophyseal ovarian axle or administered hormonal medications could also lead to mood disorders [2, 8, 38–42]. In a study that examined mental state and personality profile of infertile patients, one mental disorder at some intensity could be detected among 83.8% of women; 52% of the cases were reported to have mild or severe personality disorder [43]. In the same study, it was also revealed that in infertile patient group, depression and anxiety level were higher and mental composure was less stabile which was related with personality traits. With respect to gender, there are certain variations in mental indicators and disorders. Among infertile women, depression is reported to be more widespread; among men, on the other hand, there are a higher number of psychosomatic indicators due to suppressed anxiety [44, 45]. It was reported that among infertile men with an elevated alexithymia trait, there was higher level of experienced stress and worsened life quality [46]. Infertile women were reported to score significantly higher in the categories of psychiatric traces, hostility, cognitive dysfunction, diminished self-respect, anxiety, and depression. Among infertile men, a significant rise was observed in lower self-confidence but heightened anxiety level and somatization symptoms. Compared to women, men got higher scores in satisfaction from marriage and sexual life [47–50]. The reasons for observing more psychopathology among women can be related to assuming more responsibility and feeling of guilt, exposure to higher social pressure, and stigma [51, 52]. In one study, it was reported that 49% of infertile individuals were exposed to stigma [53]. Motherhood being a social role attributed to all women makes woman to fear infertility as a threat for marriage, which then leads to anxiety [8]. During the infertility experience, a woman having a mature personality, total self-confidence, a fulfilling bond with her spouse, and positive attitude to adoption choice can go through fewer psychological problems; on the other hand, inadequate psychological support, unsuccessful treatment interventions, low socioeconomic status, being of a foreign nationality, absence of partner support were reported to be related with heightened depression risk [46, 47]. In a noticeably significant number of studies, a critical finding showed that negative reaction of one's spouse and parents-in-law were related with higher anxiety-depression scores and lower self-esteem [20].

Mental indicators were extensively analyzed as other causes of infertility. Unexplained infertility was reported to be correlated with high anxiety level and suppressed anger; on the other hand, innate infertility was more linked with depression [54–56]. In male-related infertility cases, compared to other causes, stress level is higher in effect. In one study, it was reported that in male-caused infertility, couples avoided expressing negative emotions and it was positively linked with increased pregnancy ratios [57]. There is a correlation between mental indicators and findings and infertility itself. Findings revealed that anxiety level is a determinant for the result of infertility treatment and decision to continue the protocol [58–62]. Anxiety is also effective on patient's reaction against the possibility of losing baby after a successful treatment and pregnancy-borne complications. Also, anxiety, depression, and deteriorated marriage life are linked with unsuccessful infertility treatment. Infertility-rooted psychological problems could lead to discontinuing the treatment. It was reported that among couples not taking a second chance after a failed IVF treatment, the most decisive cause was psychological burden and incorrect prognosis [63]. Extended infertility term and unsuccessful but expensive treatment attempts were reportedly correlated with heightened depression-anxiety level. A different study indicated that rather than the length of treatment, the length of infertility was more closely associated with depression. In other studies, it was detected that compared to an average-length infertility protocol, depression levels were lower in short- and long-term infertility. Some of the reasons behind this difference are at the onset of treatment procedure, couples believe to have a baby in just a few months but as infertility period extends longer, couples may develop specific coping mechanisms and accept the situation [48–50].

8. Psychological approaches toward infertility

Psychological counseling for infertility relates to raising the awareness of individual and/or couple by spreading information and skills during diagnosis, treatment, and post-treatment stages of infertility procedure; counseling is offered by a professional specialized in the field of psychology. Patients are assisted in their decisions on treatment and can thus develop coping strategies against the devastative emotions surfaced emerging because of infertility [64]. Studies in relevant literature underlined that until the 1980s, infertility was categorized as a psychosomatic case that reflected a woman's ambivalence emotions to motherhood or unsolved conflicts with their own mothers. Hence, treatment was generically administered by psychoanalytic-oriented psychiatrists [65]. Menning [66] argued that mood changes were not the cause but rather the result of infertility. Therefore, he founded Resolve the National Infertility Association (RESOLVE) to provide emotional support for infertile individuals residing in the United States of America (USA) and climb public awareness by offering courses on infertility [66]. An increasing number of literature studies started to acknowledge psychological effects of infertility and highlighted the importance of supportive counseling interventions for those undergoing infertility treatment [66].

Psychological counselors for infertility can offer services by consulting to theoretical approaches such as psychodynamic, individual-centered, cognitive-behaviorist, or solution-focused interventions. Although the methods being employed are different from one another, all of the psychological counselors on infertility adopt a common objective in taking care of emotional well-being of the couple and when need be they strive to boost their psychological integrity and resources [67]. Responsibilities of a psychological counselor for infertility are given in **Table 1** [68–70].

As a reflection of the latest multidisciplinary medical approaches, there has been a consensus among medical community that psychological counseling should be a complementary step for the biological treatment protocol of infertile couples [71]. In psychological counseling protocol for infertility, there is a wide range of intervention types catered for the different levels of help needed among different couples. In psychological counseling for infertility, there is a myriad of counseling options such as informative and decision-making, supportive counseling, and therapeutic counseling. Informative and decision-making is the first stage of infertility counseling. This stage involves comprehensive explanations on the causes of infertility, suggested treatment options, potential expectations from the treatment, and the way treatment process could affect their everyday life [72]. At the onset of psychological counseling protocol for infertility, it is suggested to openly communicate about ideas, expectations, doubts, and worries of the clients on psychological counseling so that objectives of each session could be specified. Indeed, for many couples, this session is generally the very first meeting that they have ever had with a psychiatrist for a lifetime [70]. That is why the couple may be resistant to share their private matter with a third person and feel like being labeled. It is thus suggested that in the first session, mutual duties and responsibilities, notice on privacy, and providing a safe and supportive setting to help the patients discover and manifest their emotions toward infertility are some of the items to focus on [65]. To maintain a satisfactory session, some of the essentials are active listening, empathetic approach, adopting a respectful language toward the viewpoint of each client, identifying the meaning or importance of the problem for the client, and to make the targets achievable within the control of client. In these sessions, it is aimed to help the patients understand that most of their infertility reactions are normal and predictable, to discuss about the process toward obtaining desired solutions, to conceptualize or reinterpret the problems with solution offering methods [2].

Among the main objectives of infertility psychological counseling are providing some coping strategies to the individual and couples diagnosed with infertility,

1	Helping the couple uncover their ambivalent emotions toward being infertile
2	Helping the couple unravel their ambivalent emotions toward the projected assistive treatment methods to have a baby
3	Helping the couple cope with the complicated emotions surfacing after failed interventions
4	After nullifying the emotional limitations of the couple, helping them make a decision from a variety of options including the choice of ending the treatment
5	Helping the couple establish a more effective communication as partners on anything related to infertility
6	Helping the couple cope with ambiguity and uncontrollability phenomenon
7	Helping the couple have a clear idea on any related aspects of assisted reproductive techniques
8	Helping the couple cope with the new experience caused by pregnancy or trauma after losing the baby despite the treatment (recurrent abortus, dead birth, etc.)
9	If need be, referring mentally disordered cases to psychiatric treatment

Table 1.
Responsibilities of a psychological counselor for infertility.

emotional readiness to the treatment process, discovering the options, assisting in making a choice, and determining the effects of infertility on the individual and his/her immediate surroundings. Having recently renowned as a domain calling for professional expertise and skills, psychological counseling for infertility gives a chance to infertile individuals to seek the ways for enhancing, exploring, and clarifying their life quality and satisfaction. It also gives them a means to express infertility-related emotions such as deep misery, guilt feeling, anxiety, and explore the problem's traces on their self-perception and body image. Making sense of the emotional and physical changes undergone during treatment process is critically important in the future plans of individuals coping with infertility and to overcome the hardships they are exposed. It is thus suggested that psychological counseling for infertility that can offer the individuals a safe reserve for self-expression is quite a salient service catered for infertile individual and couples [73–77]. Psychological interventions play an important role in the treatment of infertility, in particular, for infertile patients who are not receiving medical treatment [78].

9. Conclusion

To conclude, it can be stated that infertility is a life crisis that brings with itself a number of psychological problems. Taking preventive measures upon calculating psychological problems that could affect treatment success is a critical issue to observe in providing healthcare services. During the infertility treatment process, to have some awareness on the psychological problems experienced by individuals not only helps in the adaptation of infertile individuals to infertility diagnosis and treatment procedure, but it could also lower the intensity of reactions against infertility. It is thus strongly suggested that analysis of infertile couples or individuals within the context of psychological indicators and findings should be integral to an entire infertility treatment protocol.

Acknowledgements

I offer thanks to my students.

Author details

Cicek Hocaoglu
Recep Tayyip Erdogan University Medical School, Department of Psychiatry, Rize, Turkey

*Address all correspondence to: cicekh@gmail.com

IntechOpen

References

[1] Ozçelik B, Karamustafalioğu O, Ozcelik A. Psychological and psychiatric aspects of infertility. Anadolu Psikiyatri Dergisi. 2007;**8**(2):140-148

[2] Kirca N, Pasinoglu T. Psychosocial problems during infertility treatment. Current Approaches in Psychiatry. 2013; **5**(2):162-178. DOI: 10.5455/cap.20130511

[3] Cousineau TM, Domar A. Psychological impact of infertility. Best Practice & Research: Clinical Obstetrics & Gynaecology. 2007;**21**(2):293-308

[4] Araoye MO. Epidemiology of infertility: Social problems of the infertile couples. West African Journal of Medicine. 2003;**22**(2):190-196

[5] Diriol CC, Giami A. The impact of infertility and treatment on sexual life and marital relationships: Review of the literature. Gynécologie, Obstétrique & Fertilité. 2004;**32**(7–8):624-637

[6] Ozkan M, Baysal B. Emotional distress of infertile women in Turkey. Clinical and Experimental Obstetrics & Gynecology. 2006;**33**(1):44-46

[7] Boivin J. A review of psychosocial interventions in infertility. Social Science & Medicine. 2003;**57**(12): 2325-2341

[8] Sezgin H, Hocaoglu C. Psychiatric aspects of infertility. Current Approaches in Psychiatry. 2014;**6**(2):165-184. DOI: 10.5455/cap.20131001091415

[9] Lenzi A, Lombardo F, Salacone P, Gandini L, Jannini EA. Stress, sexual dysfunctions and male infertility. Journal of Endocrinological Investigation. 2003;**26**(3):72-76

[10] Volgsten H, Skoog Svanberg A, Ekselius L, Lundkvist O, Sundström Poromaa I. Risk factors for psychiatric disorders in infertile women and men

undergoing in vitro fertilization treatment. Fertility and Sterility. 2010; **93**(4):1088-1096. DOI: 10.1016/j.fertnstert.2008.11.008

[11] Mahlstedt PP. The psychological component of infertility. Fertility and Sterility. 1985;**43**(3):335-346

[12] Onat G, Kizilkaya Beji N. Effects of infertility on gender differences in marital relationship and quality of life: A case control study of Turkish couples. European Journal of Obstetrics & Gynecology and Reproductive Biology. 2012;**165**(2):243-248. DOI: 10.1016/j.ejogrb.2012.07.033

[13] Guz H, Ozkan A, Sarisoy G, Yanik F, Yanik A. Psychiatric symptoms in Turkish infertile women. Journal of Psychosomatic Obstetrics and Gynaecology. 2003;**24**(4):267-271

[14] Matsubayashi H, Hosaka T, Shun-ichiro I, Takahiro S, Makino T. Emotional distress of infertile women in Japan. Human Reproduction. 2001; **16**(5):966-969

[15] Collins A, Freeman EW, Boxer AS, Tureck R. Perception of infertility and treatment stress in females as compared with males entering in vitro fertilization treatment. Fertility and Sterility. 1992; **57**(1):350-356

[16] Fido A, Zahid MA. Coping with infertility among Kuwaiti women: Cultural perspectives. The International Journal of Social Psychiatry. 2004; **50**(4):294-300

[17] Schmidt L. Infertility and assisted reproduction in Denmark. Epidemiology and psychosocial consequences. Danish Medical Bulletin. 2006;**53**(4):390-417

[18] Anokye R, Acheampong E, Mprah WK, Ope JO, Barivure TN. Psychosocial

effects of infertility among couples attending St. Michael's Hospital, Jachie-Pramso in the Ashanti Region of Ghana. BMC Research Notes. 2017;**10**(1):690. DOI: 10.1186/s13104-017-3008-8

[19] Matsubayashi H, Hosaka T, Izumi S, Suzuki T, Kondo A, Makino T. Increased depression and anxiety in infertile Japanese women resulting from lack of husband's support and feelings of stress. General Hospital Psychiatry. 2004; **26**(5):398-404

[20] Sezgin H, Hocaoglu C, Guvendag-Guven ES. Disability, psychiatric symptoms, and quality of life in infertile women: A cross-sectional study in Turkey. Shanghai Archives of Psychiatry. 2016;**28**(2):86-94. DOI: 10.11919/j.issn.1002-0829.216014.

[21] Khayata GM, Rizk DE, Hasan MY, Ghazal-Aswad S, Asaad MA. Factors influencing the quality of life of infertile women in United Arab Emirates. International Journal of Gynaecology and Obstetrics. 2003;**80**(2):183-188

[22] Verhaak CM, Smeenk JM, Evers AW, van Minnen A, Kremer JA, Kraaimaat FW. Predicting emotional response to unsuccessful fertility treatment: A prospective study. Journal of Behavioral Medicine. 2005;**28**(2):181-190

[23] Covington SH, Burns LH. Infertility Counselling: A Comprehensive Handbook for Clinicians. 2nd ed. New York: Cambridge University Press; 2006

[24] Klonoff-Cohen H, Natarajan L. The concerns during assisted reproductive technologies (CART) scale and pregnancy outcomes. Fertility and Sterility. 2004;**81**(4):982-988

[25] Klonoff-Cohen H, Chu E, Natarajan L, Sieber WA. Prospective study of stress among women undergoing in vitro fertilization or gamete intrafallopian transfer. Fertility and Sterility. 2001;**76**(4):675-687

[26] Zurlo MC, Cattaneo Della Volta MF, Vallone F. Predictors of quality of life and psychological health in infertile couples: The moderating role of duration of infertility. Quality of Life Research. 2018;**27**(4):945-954. DOI: 10.1007/s11136-017-1781-4

[27] Karlidere T, Bozkurt A, Yetkin S, Doruk A, Sutçigil L, Ozmenler KN, et al. Is there gender difference in infertile couples with no axis one psychiatric disorder in context of emotional symptoms, social support and sexual function? Türk Psikiyatri Dergisi. 2007; **18**(4):311-322

[28] Jedrzejczak P, Luczak-Wawrzyniak J, Szyfter J, Przewoźna J, Taszarek-Hauke G, et al. Feelings and emotions in women treated for infertility. Przegląd Lekarski. 2004;**61**(12):1334-1337

[29] Lee TY, Sun GH, Chao SC. The effect of an infertility diagnosis on treatment-related stresses. Archives of Andrology. 2001;**46**(1):67-71

[30] Jirka J, Schuatt S, Foxal JM. Lonelines and social support in infertile couples. Journal of Obstetric, Gynecologic, and Neonatal Nursing. 1996;**25**(1):55-59

[31] Monga M, Alexandrescu B, Katz SE, Stein M, Ganiats T. Impact of infertility on quality of life, marital adjusment and sexual function. Urology. 2004;**63**(1): 126-130

[32] Lee TY, Sun GH. Psychosocial response of Chinese infertile husbands and wives. Archives of Andrology. 2000;**45**(3):143-148

[33] Lee TY, Sun GH, Chao SC. The effect of an infertility diagnosis on the distress, marital and sexual satisfaction between husbands and wives in Taiwan. Human Reproduction. 2001;**16**(8):1762-1767

[34] Kamacı S. Investigation of the effect of infertility on family life in primer

infertile couples (graduation thesis). İzmir, Turkey: Ege University School of Nursing; 2003 (Turkish)

[35] Can G. Examination of anxiety and depression levels of women who applied assisted reproductive techniques (graduation thesis). İzmir, Turkey: Ege University School of Nursing; 2005 (Turkish)

[36] Chen TH, Chang SP, Cf T, Juang KD. Prevalence of depressive and anxiety disorders in an assisted reproductive technique clinic. Human Reproduction. 2004;19(10):2313-2318

[37] King RB. Subfecundity and anxiety in a nationally representative sample. Social Science & Medicine. 2003;56: 739-751

[38] De D, Roy PK, Sarkhel S. A psychological study of male, female related and unexplained infertility in Indian urban couples. Journal of Reproductive and Infant Psychology. 2017;35(4):353-364. DOI: 10.1080/02646838.2017.1315632

[39] Fido A. Emotional distress in infertile women in Kuwait. International Journal of Fertility and Women's Medicine. 2004;49(1):24-28

[40] Klemetti R, Raitanen J, Sihvo S, Saarni S, Koponen P. Infertility, mental disorders and well-being: A nationwide survey. Acta Obstetricia et Gynecologica Scandinavica. 2010;89(5):677-682. DOI: 10.3109/00016341003623746

[41] Kainz K. The role of the psychologist in the evaluation and treatment of infertility. Women's Health Issues. 2001;11(6):481-485

[42] Gulseren L, Cetinay P, Tokatlioglu B, Sarikaya OO, Gulseren S, Kurt S. Depression and anxiety levels in infertile Turkish women. The Journal of Reproductive Medicine. 2006;51(5): 421-426

[43] Lu Y, Yang L, Lu G. Mental status and personality of infertile women. Zhonghua Fu Chan Ke Za Zhi. 1995;30(1):34-37

[44] Hunt J, Monach JH. Beyond bereavement model the significance of depression for infertile women. Fertility and Sterility. 1992;58(2):1158-1163

[45] Tarlatzis I, Tarlatzis BC, Diakogiannis I, Bontis J, Lagos S, Gavriilidou D, et al. Psychosocial impacts of infertility on Greek couples. Human Reproduction. 1993;8:396-401

[46] Conrad R, Schilling G, Langenbuch M, Haidl G, Liedtke R. Alexythymia in male infertility. Human Reproduction. 2001;16:587-592

[47] Atherton F, Howel D. Psychological morbidity and the availability of assisted conception: A group comparison study. Journal of Public Health Medicine. 1995; 17:157-160

[48] Berg BJ, Wilson JF. Psychological functioning across stages of treatment of infertility. Journal of Behavioral Medicine. 1991;14:11-26

[49] Lok IH, Lee DT, Gheung LP, Chung WS, Lo WK, Haines CJ. Psychiatric morbidity amongst infertile Chinese women undergoing treatment with assisted reproductive technology and the impact of treatment failure. Gynaecologic and Obstetric Investigation. 2002;53:195-199

[50] Ramezanzadeh F, Aghssa MM, Abdinia N, Zayeri F, Khanafshar N, Shariat M, et al. A survey of relationship between anxiety, depression and duration of infertility. BMC Women's Health. 2004;4:9

[51] Whiteford LM, Gonzales L. Stigma: The hidden burden of infertility. Social Science & Medicine. 1995;40:27-36

[52] Abbey A, Andrews FM, Halman LJ. Gender's role in responses to infertility.

Psychology of Women Quarterly. 1991;
15:295-316

[53] Missmer SA, Seifer DB, Jain T.
Cultural factors contributing to health
care disparities among patients with
infertility in Midwestern United States.
Fertility and Sterility. 2011;95(6):
1943-1949. DOI: 10.1016/j.
fertnstert.2011.02.039

[54] Nachtigall RD, Becker G, Wozny M.
The effects of gender specific diagnosis
on men's and women's response to
infertility. Fertility and Sterility. 1992;
57(1):113-121

[55] Wischmann T, Stammer H, Scherg
H, Gerhard I, Verres R. Psychosocial
characteristics of infertile couples: A
study by the 'Heielberg fertility
consultation service'. Human
Reproduction. 2001;16(8):1753-1761

[56] Fassino S, Piero A, Boggio S,
Piccioni V, Garzaro L. Anxiety,
depression and anger suppression in
infertile couples: A controlled study.
Human Reproduction. 2002;17(11):
2986-2994

[57] Demyttenaere K, Bonte L, Gheldof
M, Vervaeke M, Meuleman C,
Vanderschuerem D, et al. Coping style
and depression level influence outcome
in in vitro fertilization. Fertility and
Sterility. 1998;69(6):1026-1033

[58] Demyttenaere K, Nijs P, Steeno O,
Koninckx PR, Everse-Kiebooms G.
Anxiety and conception rates in donor
insemination. Journal of Psychosomatic
Obstetrics and Gynaecology. 1988;8(1):
175-181

[59] Boivin J, Takefman JE, Tulandi T,
Brender W. Reactions to infertility
based on extent of treatment failure.
Fertility and Sterility. 1995;63(4):
801-807

[60] Boivin J, Takefman JE. Stress level
across stages of in vitro fertilization in

subsequently pregnant and nonpregnant
women. Fertility and Sterility. 1995;
64(4):802-810

[61] Smeenk JM, Verhaak CM, Eugster
A, van Minnen A, Zielhuis GA, Braat
DD. The effect of anxiety and
depression on the outcome of in-vitro
fertilization. Human Reproduction.
2001;16:1420-1423

[62] Sanders KA, Bruce NW.
Psychosocial stress and treatment
outcome following assisted reproductive
technology. Human Reproduction. 1999;
14:1656-1662

[63] Olivius C, Friden B, Borg G, Bergh
C. Why do couples discontinue in vitro
fertilization treatment? A cohort study.
Fertility and Sterility. 2004;81:258-261

[64] Applegarth LD. Individual
counseling and psychotherapy. In:
Covington SN, Burns LH, editors.
Infertility Counseling: A
Comprehensive Handbook for
Clinicians. New York: Cambridge
University Press; 2006. pp. 129-142

[65] Covington SN. Infertility counseling
in practice: A collaborative reproductive
healthcare model. In: Covington SN,
Burns LH, editors. Infertility
Counseling: A Comprehensive
Handbook for Clinicians. New York:
Cambridge University Press; 2006.
pp. 493-507

[66] Menning BE. The emotional needs
of infertile couples. Fertility and
Sterility. 1980;34:313-319

[67] Norré J, Wischmann T. The position
of the fertility counsellor in a fertility
team: A critical appraisal. Human
Fertility. 2011;14(3):154-159. DOI:
10.3109/14647273.2011.580824

[68] Read SC, Carrier ME, Boucher ME,
Whitley R, Bond S, Zelkowitz P.
Psychosocial services for couples in
infertility treatment: What do couples

really want? Patient Education and Counseling. 2014;**94**(3):390-395. DOI: 10.1016/j.pec.2013.10.025

[69] Zegers-Hochschild F, Adamson GD, Mouzon J, Ishihara O, Mansour R, Nygren K, et al. The International Committee for Monitoring Assisted Reproductive Technology (ICMART) and the World Health Organization (WHO) revised glossary on ART terminology. Fertility and Sterility. 2009;**92**(5):1520-1524. DOI: 10.1016/j.fertnstert.2009.09.009

[70] Van den Broeck U, Emery M, Wischmann T, Thorn P. Counselling in infertility: Individual, couple and group interventions. Patient Education and Counseling. 2010;**81**(3):422-428. DOI: 10.1016/j.pec.2010.10.009

[71] Van Empel IWH, Aarts JWM, Cohlen BJ, Huppelschoten DA, Laven JSE, Nelen WLDM, et al. Measuring patient-centredness, the neglected outcome in fertility care: A random multicentre validation study. Human Reproduction. 2010;**25**(10):2516-2526. DOI: 10.1093/humrep/deq219

[72] Seymenler S, Siyez MD. Infertility counseling. Current Approaches in Psychiatry. 2018;**10**(2):176-187. DOI: 10.18863/pgy.358095

[73] Mahadeen A, Mansour A, Al-Halabi J, Al Habashneh S, Kenana AB. Psychosocial wellbeing of infertile couples in Jordan. Eastern Mediterranean Health Journal. 2018; **24**(2):169-176

[74] Chow KM, Cheung MC, Cheung IK. Psychosocial interventions for infertile couples: A critical review. Journal of Clinical Nursing. 2016;**25**(15–16): 2101-2113. DOI: 10.1111/jocn.13361

[75] Denton J, Monach J, Pacey A. Infertility and assisted reproduction: Counselling and psychosocial aspects. Human Fertility (Cambridge, England). 2013;**16**(1):1. DOI: 10.3109/14647273.2013.781335

[76] Karaca A, Unsal G. Psychosocial problems and coping strategies among Turkish women with infertility. Asian Nursing Research (Korean Society of Nursing Science). 2015;**9**(3):243-250. DOI: 10.1016/j.anr.2015.04.007

[77] Malina A, Błaszkiewicz A, Owczarz U. Psychosocial aspects of infertility and its treatment. Ginekologia Polska. 2016; **87**(7):527-531. DOI: 10.5603/GP.2016.0038

[78] Dancet EA, D'Hooghe TM, Spiessens C, Sermeus W, De Neubourg D, Karel N, et al. Quality indicators for all dimensions of infertility care quality: Consensus between professionals and patients. Human Reproduction. 2013; **28**(6):1584-1597. DOI: 10.1093/humrep/det056

www.ingramcontent.com/pod-product-compliance
Lightning Source LLC
Chambersburg PA
CBHW081238190326
41458CB00016B/5832